Intermitter

Women Over 50

The Ultimate Guide for a Natural

Approach to Weight Loss and Looking

Younger, Formulated for Mature

Women

Megan Whiteley

Table of Contents

Introduction

Thank you for your purchase of *Intermittent Fasting for Women over 50: The Ultimate Guide for a Natural Approach to Weight Loss and Looking Younger, Formulated for Mature Women.*

The goal of this book is to acquaint women with the things they can expect from their bodies, their dietary regimens, their metabolisms, and their energy levels at a certain point in life. Our bodies aren't as elastic or as resilient as they once were, but with the proper knowledge to hand, that doesn't need to be a bad thing!

With intermittent fasting, you will find that the regimen equips your body to handle the foods you're putting into it without accumulating excess stores of fat that your body can't or won't use for long periods of time. You'll be preparing your body to do the most it can with what you give it and you'll be focusing on taking in wholesome, healthful foods without depriving yourself of flavor, carbohydrates, fats, or natural sugars.

In moderate amounts and when taken on at precise points throughout the day and the week, you will find that your body processes foods in a much more predictable manner, making your energy levels feel higher than they have on any other regimen. You'll feel great between your meals, you won't suffer through your fasts, and you'll have the energy to do all the things that make life most enjoyable and worth living!

Too many women who reach this mature age are left to feel that their best years are behind them and that things are on a downward slope. By taking care of our bodies and giving them the things they crave and by understanding our internal processes and helping them to do what they do best, many of us will find that we feel just as well as we ever have, if not better!

We know that when it comes to books on lifestyles and healthful regimens, you have countless choices. Thank you very much for choosing this book to guide you in your new journey toward health and wellness. Every effort was made to ensure that the information in this book was brought to you with utmost clarity and validity.

Please enjoy!

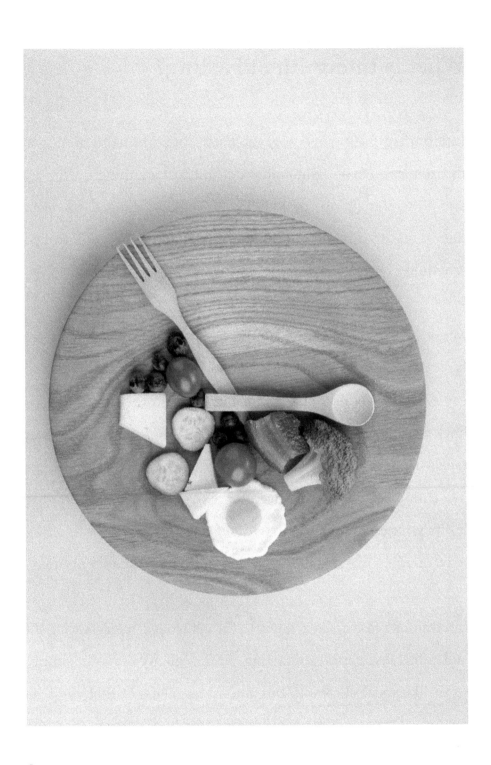

What is Intermittent Fasting?

Intermittent fasting is one of the most popular dieting trends at the moment. It's a regimen that doesn't cost anything to employ and it's something that helps countless dieters to keep themselves to a regimen of lower intake and a more controlled schedule in between meals.

Many of us feel like we're tethered to the mealtimes that we typically keep and we feel like we're interrupted by the need to eat every few hours throughout the day. However, some of us have taken to skipping meals without making sure that our other meals are nutritionally sound and this can lead us to do things like eating overly large meals after a skipped meal or indulging in the wrong kinds of foods without realizing what we're doing to our bodies, our metabolisms, and our overall quality of life.

Intermittent fasting is a regimen of controlled meal placement and controlled periods of fasting. At first glance, it might simply seem like meal skipping, but the added element that can't be missed or forgotten is ensuring that our bodies are getting the nourishment they require throughout each day, even on the days when we've chosen not to eat anything.

The core concept of intermittent fasting doesn't dictate what you should or should not be eating, but it does dictate the intervals at which you eat and at which you fast. This book will, however, make recommendations for the best and worst foods to eat while you're doing intermittent fasting to ensure that you're getting the absolute most out of your dietary regimen.

In the ancient history of mankind, all the way up through the 19th century, and even into the 20th, you will see evidence of food scarcity that makes today's food availability seem utterly astonishing. Even as recently as the 1950s, taking your entire family out to eat at a restaurant was a big deal that didn't occur nearly as often as it does today. Some of the readers of this book will remember dressing up to go out anywhere, as it was an occasion.

For many depressed areas, food scarcity is still an issue, but by and large, you will find that no modern dieter is faced with a shortage of available foods. Because of the amount of food that is available to us on demand at any time of day, we're often taking on far more calories than we realistically needs, and our bodies are struggling to find places to store all the excess fat created as a result of that overly-generous intake.

With intermittent fasting, you're cutting down your calorie intake by shaving off a meal here and there throughout your week and you're giving your body the chance to adapt and boost its hormone production that will allow you to access and break down those stores of fat your body has created over the years. By doing this, you'll find that your body is creating energy, even when you have not eaten recently.

Because your body will be getting accustomed to this method of living and this means of procuring energy, you'll find that you have more energy on a more consistent basis throughout the day. Because your body has onboard stores of energy that it can now access, you won't experience those midday slumps or crashes. You won't feel faint after several hours of not eating, because your body is still getting everything it needs from those stores!

As you may have already deduced, there is a very fortunate result of your body making use of those fat stores: weight loss!

As that fat is burned and used by your body, you'll notice that you're losing pounds and inches in places that you never even thought possible! That stubborn bit right around the waist that seemed to resist even the hardest core workouts will slip away quietly while you fast and you might even find those areas on the upper arms shrinking before you know it as well.

While these stubborn, problematic areas might not be the first to go, your body will have no option but to *eventually* make use of those fat stores. No fat cell is too stubborn to be swept away and used by your body when you're on a strict and steady regimen of intermittent fasting!

Why Does it Help?

Choosing to fast at intermittent periods throughout your week can give you an advantage that allows your metabolism to change for the better, allows you to cut down your intake throughout the week, and it can help you to feel your best. Throughout history and cultures all across the globe, you will see references to and instances of fasting. This is influenced by a number of factors throughout history, but the chief one is the scarcity of food.

It just so happens that our bodies are accustomed to the periodic scarcity of food and can thrive on it more than we may previously have believed. When we give our body intermittent periods of food scarcity, our bodies are forced to sustain themselves on the fat stores that our bodies have accumulated over the years.

Excess glucose that is taken on by the body is stored as fat to be used later. This is the mechanism that allowed humankind to survive those periodic stages of food scarcity and our bodies are still operating in that same way. You might notice that your body has some stores of fat that it has kept around a little longer than you might like. That's because your body is waiting for its perfect opportunity to put those stores to use! By doing intermittent fasting, you give your body every opportunity to put those stores to use and to subsist off of them, without depriving your body of the essential nutrients it needs in order to thrive and survive.

By making sure that the meals you eat are healthy, wholesome, and packed with all the right things, you're making sure that your body isn't simply starving during the times when you're not eating. It's got plenty of energy to use with the stores of fat in your body, and it's got all the nutrients from the supplements and the wholesome foods you're eating.

The hormonal changes in your body are what allow you to get access to those stores of fat and to break them down for energy. In addition to this, you will find that your sensitivity to insulin will improve. If you have difficulties with your insulin tolerance or the stability of your blood sugar levels, you might find that doing intermittent fasting is helpful for this.

Many people who have trouble with their blood sugar regularity will find they have trouble with keeping themselves from crashing in the early afternoon. People who struggle with that might find that they have trouble staying full until their next meal and may even feel a little bit of lightheadedness or mood swings between meals. This could be the indication of something a little more serious depending on how difficult it is for you to sustain yourself between mealtimes, so be sure that your doctor is checking your A1C for evidence of diabetes.

If you have found that you do have type II diabetes that developed as a result of certain eating habits, it is something that can typically be reversed with the help of a structured diet that contains more of the foods your body needs in order to survive and less of the foods that interfere with your body's use of insulin. In such cases, however, you will want to ensure that you are taking on the right foods in the right quantities to hold you over between meals, meaning you might need to start your fasting on a much more stringent and abbreviated timeline with the help of your doctor.

Many people who are working to turn around their diabetes have found that, with a specially-planned regimen, they were able to work toward an intermittent fasting schedule while they worked to improve their diabetes or insulin sensitivity. By filling your body with 2,000 or fewer calories of wholesome, nutritious, low-glycemic foods, you might find that your condition will improve and your ability to stabilize your blood sugar for several hours at a time will improve along with that, allowing you to branch out to and get onto an intermittent fasting regimen that works for you!

Why is This Method Ideal for Women over 50?

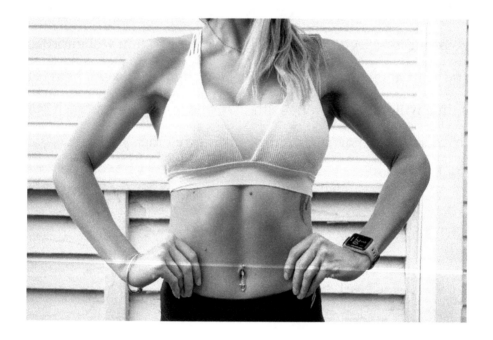

Once we age beyond 50 years, our bodies start to change in the ways they handle certain things. Sugar, fat, and diets as a whole. You might find that things you could eat with no issue as recently as five years ago, are suddenly giving you heartburn or causing you to have troubles when it's time to go to the restroom. For many of this, it strikes us as a cruel aspect of reality and it seems like we're moving past the things that we enjoy in life and that we're relegated to less interesting meals.

While this is a negative frame of mind, I completely understand it and you're entitled to feel that way at first. It is important to know, however, that your metabolism and your body are simply shifting into a different phase and that you've got a lot of other things going on, especially hormone-wise. You will find that with things like menopause and certain other aspects of the aging process are the reasons we have to adjust a lot of things. You might be surprised to learn that the things you eat do have a bearing on how you're feeling and they do have a bearing on how quickly and easily your body adapts to those changes. I'm not saying they're solely responsible, simply that the fuel you're giving your body does make a difference.

With intermittent fasting, your focus is not only on the structure you use for your meal consumption but also on ensuring that your body is getting all of the whole nutrients it needs in order to function properly while you're eating. If you commit to doing the intermittent fasting regimen, you must also commit to making sure that your meals contain all the right things to sustain you, to activate the right hormone production in your body, and the supplemental nutrition you will need in order to make the very most of the time your body is spending breaking down the fat stores in your body for crucial nutrition and energy.

While your body is making these adjustments in the way it's continuing to regenerate cells for hair, skin, organs, etc., it is making use of the food you're giving it in order to do those things. If you're able to provide your body with the ideal balance of macronutrients (fat, protein, and carbohydrates) from ideal and nourishing sources, you will find that your body simply thrives on what it's been given. You will find that the processes in your body—everything from the simple stuff like sleeping to the more complex stuff like organ health—will continue on with more ease.

Some women in this age group have found themselves grappling with things that were never a problem for them before. Some women find that in spite of the fact that they were carrying on through their days while feeling like they could fall asleep standing up and any moment, they are completely unable to sleep when the time finally comes for them to hang up their hats for the day. Some women find that around the time they would typically be menstruating, their bodies are throwing curveballs at them that are simply impossible to anticipate. Some women find that their digestive system simply won't process things in the way that it once did.

Our bodies tend to need a much higher balance of things like vitamins, minerals, fiber, and things that can tend to be forgotten in the everyday diet unless you've spent a lot of time being very health-conscious. Many of us have simply been busy living our lives, minding what we eat, exercising when we can, without breaking down the daily values and percentages of everything we eat to find out what works best. Most of us haven't conducted our diets using the scientific method, figuring out what measures of certain nutrients are better than others.

While intermittent fasting doesn't go that far, it can certainly feel like that in the beginning, and it is crucial that you be on lookout for the changes in your body and your overall wellness to ensure that you're making changes for the better and that your body is gaining benefits from the methods and foods you're using from day to day.

For women our age, it can seem like there are just a lot of things going on in our bodies all at once and you really wouldn't be wrong in assuming that. Where you might be mistaken in your assumption, however, is that it doesn't need to be the end of the world and it doesn't have to be very hard to turn the ship around. You have a lot of life ahead of you and you have a lot left to do here with life, family, goals, and all the things you have worked so hard for in your life.

Life is meant to be enjoyed and that does not change, no matter what age you've reached. Intermittent fasting is here to give you the tools to make life enjoyable so you can continue to do what makes life worth living without having to suffer at the hands of changing bodily processes and hormone outputs!

Converting Your Body Fat

As has been mentioned in other sections of this book, your body is going to be making use of the fat that's in your body. If you don't have a good deal of excess body fat to use to hold you over during your fasts, not to worry! Simply ensure that your intake contains plenty of healthy fats for your body to use and that your nutrition is sound! Let's talk about this subject in a little bit more detail, though, shall we?

In most other diets and with most exercise and weight loss regimens, you will find that the goal is to burn the fat and purge it from your body. While this is all well and good, it does not result in a *metabolic reset*, which we will be covering in the next section of this chapter. Your body simply burns the fat without processing it or making use of it and the fat is purged from your body through the urine. Not a pleasant fact, but a fact nonetheless.

If you are someone who has a significant amount of excess fat in your body, then you should take a look at your body and give yourself a new frame of mind regarding the bits of "extra." The extra bodyweight that is on you at this moment should not be considered "excess" and it shouldn't be considered something that is useless and to be done away with at the earliest convenience.

Instead, I put it to you at this moment that your body has stored potential energy for you and that you now have that much fuel to help you to get through a new dietary regimen without feeling like you're starving or depriving yourself of anything. The stores of fat in your body are quite literally going to be the fuel that keeps you going while you're fasting. If you'd like, you can look at it as "I'm not even fasting, I'm just dipping into the fuel savings account that my body has set up and filled for me over the years!"

This might sound silly at first, but that little shift in mindset can do wonders for the feeling of deprivation or punishment that often comes with the diet and a new dietary regimen, especially one that requires you to refrain from eating for long periods of time. In fact, the reason many women find themselves shying away from certain dietary regimens or failing to stay committed to them is because some of them are downright medieval in the way they make women feel about their bodies and their reasons to stay committed to those regimens.

Your reasons for making use of your body's fat stores and your reasons for wanting a more structured approach to your mealtimes are your *own* reasons and they are valid, whatever they are. However, it can put a damper on things to feel like the regimen you're on doesn't allow you to go out with friends, to enjoy anything, or to host or join parties.

As I mentioned in the previous section, life is for living and if your dietary regimen dictates that you bring a non-dairy cheesecake to a cookout, you might find that you're less likely to enjoy it around all that other food, and you might find yourself less inclined to even continue the regimen after no one else enjoyed that "cheesecake" either!

This isn't a rip on people who have committed to and enjoy a dairy-free lifestyle, it is only to illustrate that we become accustomed to certain tastes and foods and if there is no room to fit any of those things into your regimen from time to time, you might be less inclined to endure it or deal with it for as long as you might need to in order to reach those loftier goals.

What's even more, because there is no metabolic reset in those dietary programs or regimens, you will often find that the weight just comes right back at the earliest possible convenience! This yo-yo effect can make it impossible to what to stick with any regimen at all because so many of us go into diets with a very temporary mindset.

We go into these diets thinking, "I'm going to lose these 35 pounds and then I can go back to living my life the way I want!" Because of this, there's no change in the way our bodies metabolize and deal with the nutrients we give them and the fat stores come right back. And that's only in the cases when those diets were successful in breaking down those fat stores in the first place!

The ideal answer is to *convert* the fat in your body into fuel, to burn it off while getting that stored energy out of it, to burn off the most stubborn areas, and to enjoy life *while you're doing it!* This will allow you to enjoy life and your regimen, and it will allow your body to make the necessary changes to keep you from needing to bounce around from regimen to regimen, hoping for something that will make you look and feel the way you wish to each and every day!

Metabolic Reset

Now, you've probably heard of regimens talking about the fact that they "reset your metabolism," but what does that mean? Does that mean that, by eating this way, I will suddenly have the metabolism that I had in high school? It absolutely does *not* mean that, but oh what a world we'd have ahead of us if it did!

No, what it *does* mean, however, is that we're giving your metabolism the chance to handle what you're throwing at it without it feeling that it needs to take any of the nutrients you're ingesting and relegate them to the fat stores in your body. By setting up your body to digest on a specific schedule, by giving your body all the right nutrients, by nourishing your body completely and settling into this regimen, you are giving your body a purpose to assign to those stores of fat and to make use of anything inside it before storing anything new.

Studies have found that the act of cutting down one's intake and fasting on a specific schedule can have a drastic impact on the way in which your body handles the food you ingest. The speed at which it processes your food and the readiness with which it purges the portions of that food it doesn't use will increase.

In addition to this, getting a metabolic reset means that your overall digestive health and metabolic health will be improved as well. You will find it easier to handle and digest the occasional indulgence in the foods that aren't as wholesome, but which we enjoy from time to time. Your body becomes more able to discern the things it should use and keep and the things that it should simply purge from the body over time.

I can't neglect to mention the very integral part of this: the hormones. As I've mentioned previously, your body will be producing hormones like the Human Growth Hormone and insulin on more convenient scales and schedules to benefit your body. When your body is making and using these hormones properly, you will find that digestion, weight loss, and life, in general, are far more pleasant. The Human Growth Hormone is something that can greatly aid in the access and breakdown of fat stores in the body, so this is more or less the key to your weight loss when using the intermittent fasting regimen to your advantage.

Boosting Cellular Health

When your body takes on nutrients and breaks them down for energy, your body makes use of that energy and those nutrients to do everything it has to do. There are significantly more processes going on in our bodies to keep us going than we may even realize. Everything seems so automatic in our bodies that it can escape our thinking to consider them.

If you're following the food is fuel analogy, you can think of your body like a four-cylinder engine that runs very well on premium fuel. German engineering purrs like a kitten when you really get it going, and it requires good upkeep and a little bit of babying here and there. Eating things like fast food that is packed with sodium and fillers can have the comparable effects on your body as that engine would experience when given diesel fuel. It's not a pretty picture and the car can't be expected to operate as well or as cleanly without any issues, can it? You can't pour vodka into a lawnmower and expect it to run!

Cells count on the fuel you give it in order to restore themselves, protein in particular. Your cells regenerate on a constant basis, and you've likely heard that every seven years, your body has a completely different set of cells than it did in the previous seven. In order for those cells to regenerate, renew, and reproduce, we need to give them essential amino acids, fatty acids, proteins, minerals, vitamins, and wholesome nutrients that allow them to do what they do best without any interference from us or from junky foods.

Foods that contain fillers, sodium and nutrients we cannot break down and use are aptly called junk foods. They might fill us up, they might satisfy, they might make us feel good for a short period of time, but our bodies pack up the components of those foods into lumpy little boxes and places squarely on your hips until such time as your body can get around to using it for *something* or simply purging it!

Taking on foods of this kind with any sort of regularity is you telling your cells "this is the fuel you get, so make it work." Your cells then have to use those nutrients to the best of their ability and they work really hard to regenerate with what you've given them. I don't know about you, but I would much rather have cells built with the nutrients from a chicken breast than I would from a candy bar. There's something about that perspective that simply lights a fire under me to do better about the fuel I'm giving my cells.

If this strikes a chord with you, think about saying a little speech to yourself at the beginning of your meals. Look over your food and say, "this is going into my body and my body will be using this food in order to determine the direction my health is ultimately going in."

Every single meal you eat counts as a step toward or away from your health goals, and if you're having meals that are packed with nutrients your body can reliably use for health, then you know you're going in the right direction. Foods with healthy fats, foods with protein, foods without preservatives and non-digestible additives, foods with fiber, foods with vitamins and minerals, and foods that make you *feel good* should be your primary concern when you're looking to boost your cellular health.

Intermittent Fasting and You

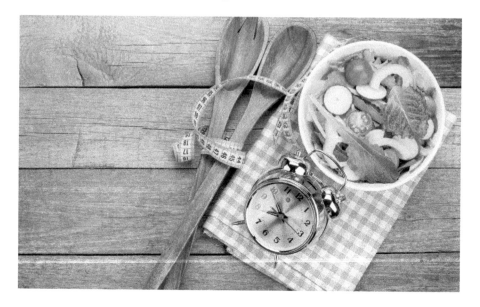

The Pros of Intermittent Fasting

It actively promotes health.

The foods that you're encouraged to eat in this book are nutritious foods, but you might not find that the other sources you're looking to are encouraging this. Intermittent fasting, as a regimen, does not dictate that you change the foods you eat, but in spite of this, many people experience benefits for their health simply because of the weight loss that occurs and the schedule that your body can predict. As it turns out, eating on a particular schedule that your body can anticipate can allow your body to "warm up" before you eat, allowing it to break down and use those foods with more ease.

Weight loss is almost inevitable.

Because you're cutting out a meal here and there, you will find that your body is utilizing your excess fat stores during the times when you would normally be eating. Even in cases when you're not necessarily cutting out calories, your body is still using those stores of fat in your body to tide it over when you would typically be eating a meal! If you're fasting during breakfast one day and your body has released the hormones that allow your body to make use of that fat, your body will do so on its own during that "skipped" meal! This results in the loss of fat stores in *any* event!

Your brain function can actually increase.

Many people who have done intermittent fasting have found that their mental processes are actually clearer than they were before they begun to fast. Because the brain produces hormones in order to function and because hormone function is overall increased and improved, you will find that your abilities to think in a straight line and to recall things might actually increase. You might find it easier to deal with the day to day and you might find that you aren't thinking in circles or forgetting things as much as you once were!

Stubborn fat that is hard to get rid of will disappear.

All of us have at least one area in our body that is just a little bit softer than other areas, and which doesn't seem to respond to even the most intense workouts we do from time to time. Many of us have a spot that we wish we could hide with a slimmer or that we just prefer no one looks at or photographs. When we start doing intermittent fasting, that fat becomes an onboard fuel source that our bodies can break down and use. Once the other fats in your body are used, your system will tap into those areas and make use of the fat that's stored there!

You don't *technically* **need to change anything about how you eat.**

If you decide to continue researching this topic beyond the pages of this book, you will find that a lot of blogs, posts, and advertisements boast that you simply don't need to change *anything* about the foods you eat in order to lose weight! While it is true that even if you keep eating what you're currently eating and simply change your schedule around, you will lose weight and your body will make use of the excess fat that is stored in it.

37

However, if you make changes to ensure that your body is getting whole, nutritious, and delicious foods when you're in periods of eating, you will look and feel better that much faster.

It's very straightforward.

Once you choose and work up to a fasting regimen that works for you, there is no need to look into or try others. If you've found a schedule that allows you to eat at the times that are most convenient for you, there really isn't too much more that you need to know in order to start having success with it! There aren't a lot of changes, there aren't a lot of variations that you really need to watch or take into account with your day to day. You simply need to a) make sure that the food you're eating is nutritious b) make sure that you're eating enough c) don't binge and d) eat when you're supposed to. Bing, bang, boom. You're intermittent fasting with the best of them and you're getting results!

Since your meals will typically be slightly larger, you will feel full when you're done eating, which is rare for a diet.

As has been mentioned, you want to refrain from binging or eating large amounts of food while you're on your breaks between fasts. However, because you will need a good number of nutrients for when you're fasting, you will find that your meals don't diminish in size at all between fasts. This allows you to eat an amount that is *satisfactory* for you, which is not typical of diets. On most dietary regimens, your intake is cut down drastically and you're required to eat less and less while you lose weight, forcing your body to stop telling you it's hungry after a while, even though you're still feeding it less than it needs in order to maintain its weight.

Get a break from the typical diet mentality.

You will find that most diets rely on you paring down the amount that you are eating and just grin and bear it until you've lost enough to stop. There is a mentality of deprivation, of enduring, and of "thinking thin." With intermittent fasting, the goal is to shift your metabolism into a mode of healthful survival and to keep you looking and feeling better with each passing day. It is not *required* of you to make drastic changes to the things that you eat and it is not *required* of you that you follow anyone's patterns but your own. You can find the method that works most ideally for you and you can roll with it until you feel like you've made a dramatic and positive impact on your body and on your health.

The lessening of inflammation.

The body isn't given a lot of downtime between meals and it's busy digesting the foods that we give it while we're eating normally. A lot of people don't realize that the foods they're eating are causing a bit of inflammation in the gut and in the body that cause things like back pain, lowered kidney function, stomach aches, bloating, and a whole host of other symptoms we've chalked up to other reasons. However, when you give your body a "break" from digesting foods and you allow your body to simply break down and use the fat it's already mostly digested, your body can repair and cut down that inflammation in your body. You might even figure out some of the foods that cause that inflammation so you can reduce or eliminate it!

Regulation of your body's hormones.

The hormone in the digestive system and even in the brain are created and utilized throughout the body in the measures that they're meant to when you're giving your body the opportunity to change the mass of fat within it. You would be shocked to learn how much of an effect excess fat can have on the body's internal processes and how good it feels to have those processes alleviated with the gradual—yet dramatic—removal of that fat. Your body's hormones will regulate over time and you will feel a better balance within you than you may have thought possible!

A healthy metabolism that can handle curveballs in the long run.

When your metabolism is operating at peak and ideal levels, you can have the occasional slice of cake or big meal out with friends without completely spinning yourself off course. Some diets are conducted on such a fine balance that one big meal can wreck weeks of progress and can make it completely impossible to get started again. There is one diet that relies on the deprivation of calories to almost nil for weeks at a time, which relies on a sort of

41

metabolic momentum to keep progress going. One misstep and weight loss is stalled for several days until you can build that momentum back up again! With intermittent fasting, you simply hop back to it as soon as you're done with that variation, and you'll find your progress will continue to roll right along!

Very easy to follow.

You don't need any pesky apps, no weekly weigh-ins, no complex meal tracking, and no beating yourself up for any little mistake that you make. You simply pick a schedule that works for you, write it into your calendar if that helps you to stay informed of your schedule, and eat when you're supposed to. There doesn't need to be much more to it than that if that is the sort of simplicity that you enjoy in a regimen.

No hard limits on nutrient intake.

If you're feeling hungrier one day than another, simply eat a little bit more without overdoing it. Because there are no numbers and hard limits for you to follow on every macronutrient, you don't need to write anything down if you don't wish to do so. You don't need to punish yourself for a little extra of something if you feel like your body needs it that day. This regimen is about giving your body what it needs so it can thrive on what it has right now. That's all there is to it!

No calorie counting.

While it's not advised to eat more than you need in one day, you don't need to hold yourself to any one limit on your calorie intake. You can simply have a meal that you enjoy, which is made up of foods that benefit your body, and move on with your day. Dieting is a very small part of your life. What you eat doesn't need to rule your life and you have far more important things to concern yourself with, so we don't demand that you devote more time and attention than you reasonably have for this regimen.

The Cons of Intermittent Fasting

If you're not careful about your schedule, your fasts could coincide with your mealtimes with friends and family.

There can be moments when you're doing intermittent fasting that your fasts end up colliding with some other engagement that is conducted over food. (Seriously, you're never as shocked by how much of our lives involve food until you're worried about eating less of it.) In such cases, you might find that you have to reschedule the gathering or your fast. Rescheduling your fast might be uncomfortable for you, especially if you're not completely established on it yet, but there is *always* a solution!

In the beginning, you may feel sluggish.

When you're getting used to how intermittent fasting affects your body and how to eat in order to sustain yourself, you might find that your body doesn't know *what* is going on. It's not like you can tell your body, "listen, it's going to get better, so stop feeling so crummy right now until you get food again." You might find that you feel completely sluggish or dead tired in the middle of your first few fasts. If you find that this happens, try to hydrate a little bit more and fill in with the tips and tricks later in this book to get you through those rougher periods.

In the beginning, you might have mood swings.

We've all been there. We've all been a little too long without a meal and found ourselves getting snippy at every little thing that pops across our path to inconvenience us or to get in between us and the food we so desperately feel we need. In these instances, it's a great idea to take a minute, take some deep breaths, and tell yourself that it's the hunger that's getting to you. It can take a lot of mental and emotional fortitude to stop ourselves from saying something we really don't mean when we're starving, but you will find that taking just an extra minute or two before we respond can make a world of difference.

In the beginning, you might find yourself "slumping" a little more than usual.

It's definitely possible to feel a midday crash when you're doing your first few fasts. You might find that in addition to the sudden and dramatic lack of energy in your body, you just feel a lot less

45

happy than you typically do. This is not an uncommon occurrence when you're first starting out with your fasting. It's not a pleasant circumstance, but if you can get yourself through that initial hurdle, you will find that your hormones (stress and sadness hormones as well) will regulate and you won't have nearly as much difficulty with your mindset.

It can be hard not to binge when coming off of a fast.

This really is a hard urge to overcome when you feel like you're starving to death after a fast. You might feel like it's impossible not to swallow your next meal whole or like it's impossible not to want to carbo-load and while that's not uncommon, I do have to recommend against it for your health. As counter-intuitive as it might seem, try to pace yourself when you're eating that first meal after a fast. Try to stretch it out so it takes you about twenty minutes to finish the meal. Set the fork down in between bites and perhaps have an engaging conversation or read something fascinating while you eat. This can help you to distract yourself from the overwhelming need to eat and you will often find that your body will register that you are full much more readily.

If you're trying to cut carbs without increasing fiber, you may have trouble "going."

Many people have this trouble with keto as well. If you are cutting down on carbohydrates, upping your healthy fat intake, and upping your protein intake without increasing your fiber, you might find it to be an uphill struggle to achieve digestive regularity. If you're having trouble even though it seems like you are eating enough vegetables and fruits to aid in things, consider a water-soluble fiber powder supplement that will help you to move things along. If issue with this persist, do speak with your doctor about the best way to proceed.

Weight loss doesn't always manifest right away.

During the first weeks of intermittent fasting, your body will be acclimating to a *lot* of changes and it might take some time for it to switch everything over so your body can make use of those stores of fat in your body. Especially if you're not making a decrease in the amount of food you're taking on from day to day or the quality of that food, you might feel a little stuck in the beginning. Don't let this scare you away!

It's not for everyone, and it might chase you away.

The mood swings, the slumps, the crashes, the feeling of deprivation, and the difficulty of acclimating to a system like this simply may not be for you. There is nothing wrong with that at all and, if it doesn't work, then there's no reason to keep pushing it on yourself! The goal of intermittent fasting is happier, healthier people and if this just doesn't happen to be the right means for you to achieve that, then so be it. There is something out there that suits your individual needs and the fact that you're making a commitment to your health and wellness is a great step in itself and I wish you the best in finding the right regimen for you and your family.

Could conflict with medications.

Not eating for long periods of time can conflict with medications, particularly if they're meant to be taken with food. Be sure to speak with your doctor about the regimen you're considering and the schedule on which you're thinking of fasting. Ensure that your doctor doesn't have any alternative recommendations to line up with your health and your medicines before committing to *any* regimen, regardless of types. Medications are an added variable that many don't consider before trying something new and with something as crucial as your diet, you really should have all the facts in your arsenal first.

The severe hunger one may feel in the beginning can be too much of a hurdle to overcome for some.

In some cases, the hunger is just something that you can't get past. For people who are just starting out, it's recommended to make concessions when it's absolutely necessary as a sort of "training wheels" until you really hit your stride with the schedule and regimen that you feel would work best for you. If that doesn't happen for you, even after several honest and earnest attempts to do so, then it might be something that isn't for you. Give it your best to adapt, but if it's not for you, then there's nothing wrong with that and you may simply need a different regimen!

You might feel a drop in your willingness or ability to be active for some time in the beginning.

It's hard enough to get up the gumption to run off to the gym to do lots of strenuous activity. It's even harder when you have not eaten in several hours and it's even harder to want to exert yourself if you feel like you're already fighting to get even enough energy to get through work past three in the afternoon. Allow yourself a period of adjustment before you commit to exercise and, when you do work exercise back into your regimen, try to place it during times when you are eating so your body is taking on as much fuel as possible to help with that workout. You should also increase your protein intake if you're working out to allow your muscles to recuperate and renew after those workouts.

Could be hard to maintain for an extended period of time.

Sometimes life changes or shifts, and sometimes something that you thought would just be your new lifestyle needs to be something temporary. With intermittent fasting, it really could go either way. The important thing is to listen to your body and do what it's telling you to do. It's crucial to let something run its course and not to belabor it if you've gotten all that you possibly can get from it. If you've lost lots of weight, you've achieved your goals, and you simply don't feel as good as you once did while doing the regimen, discontinue the regimen and simply keep your eating habits healthy and stable and that should serve you well from there on out!

The Adjustment Period

In the very beginning, your body is going through kind of a lot all at once. Many processes that are going on internally are happening all at once and it may take some of them a little bit of extra time to catch up when you might not have thought that would be the case. If you get to the end of your first fast and you feel like you might just throw your hands up in the air, devour an entire pizza, and take a nap on the couch before resuming your normal eating activities and never looking at intermittent fasting again, I'm sure no one would blame you.

Fasting can feel like it just *sucks* in the very beginning and you might find yourself feeling like it's just not worth it to keep going. *However*, if you're able to fight through those urges, take the time to have a healthy, wholesome meal at the end of your fast, fill in with some healthy snacks here and there, and give your body all that it needs to thrive in between fasts, you might find that the next one doesn't go over like a lead balloon! You might find that the simple act of waiting it out and giving your body more of the good stuff was enough to keep everything going in just the right direction.

The adjustment to fasting is very rarely going to be a completely fast and easy process that you'll get through with no fuss and no muss. You will often find that you need to find reasons to continue, to find things that make the fasts a little bit easier to get through, or things that you can eat between fasts that make them a little bit easier to handle. For some people, there is no right answer except to find a different regimen, but I want you to know that anyone who knows anything about intermittent fasting will applaud you for giving yourself the chance to make those adjustments and to get through that initial, very upsetting period.

It's crucial in the beginning of your diet to make sure that you're supported well by the people around you, to make sure that you have your mindset clear as to why you're doing this, and that you are doing things to enrich your life *around the diet*. So many of us, when we're getting committed to a new regimen, will just kind of drop everything while we're getting started, leaving us plenty of time to dwell on the fact that we're not eating all the things we wish we were eating, and to wonder if weight loss really is worth all of this hullaballoo. I can assure you that it *is* worth the hullaballoo and you will feel that this is more accurate when the things that you're doing around the diet are things that you enjoy.

If you are retired and you are at home or doing very little while you're in the middle of your very first fast, or even the first few fasts, you might find them much harder to get through. Distraction is a cruel mistress when you're fasting. Eating out of boredom is a huge problem for millions of people across the world, especially those who are at home (where all their food is) or when we're not doing something that is particularly engaging or entertaining.

If you do find yourself trying to work through the hunger and having no luck pushing that distraction out of your mind, take a little walk. A little 15-minute walk is a great way to help you center your mind on the tasks that you would rather be doing, and it's a great way to pass a little bit of time while being somewhat active as well!

After you've been doing intermittent fasting for a while and you get a little bit more comfortable with your fasting periods, you will find that you need fewer and fewer coping mechanisms and that you can simply live your life as you normally would, regardless of the fasting that's happening concurrently. This is the goal, as you want to be able to live your life around the regimen without it interfering in anything!

What to Eat

Berries.

Berries are very healthy, incredibly flavorful, and much lower in calories and sugar than you might think! Their tart sweetness can really bring a smoothie to life and they make an absolutely delicious snack on their own without any help from things like cream or sugar.

Cruciferous vegetables.

These are the vegetables like cabbage, Brussels sprouts, broccoli, and cauliflower. These are wonderful additions to your diet because they're packed with vital nutrients and with fiber that your body will love and use with a quickness!

Eggs.

Eggs are such a great addition to your diet because they're packed to the gills with protein, you can do just about anything with them, they're easy to prepare, they travel well if you hard boil them, and they can pair with just about anything. They're a great protein source for salads, and they're good on their own as well.

Fish.

Fish are a wonderful source of protein and healthy fats. White fish, in particular, is typically very lean, but fish like salmon that have a little bit of color in them are packed with protein, fats, and oils that are great for you. They're good for brain and heart health, and there's a huge array of delicious things you can do with them.

Healthy starches like certain potatoes (with skins!)

Red potatoes, in particular, are perfectly fine to eat, even if you're trying to lose weight because your body can use those carbs for fuel and the skins are packed with minerals that your body will enjoy. A little bit of potato here and there can do good things for your nutrition, but they are also a great way to feel like you're getting a little more of those fun foods that you should cut back on.

57

Legumes.

Beans, beans, the magical fruit. They're packed with protein and the starch in them just makes them stick to your ribs without making you pay for it later. They're wonderful in soups, salads, and just about any other meal of the day that you're looking to fill out. By adding beans to your regimen, you might find that your meals stick with you a little bit longer and leave you feeling more satisfied than you thought possible.

Nuts.

I know you've heard people talking about how a handful of almonds makes a great snack and if you're anything like me, you've always had kind of a hard time believing it. Nuts, as it turns out, have a good deal of their own healthy fats in them that your body can use to get through those rough patches and, while they not be the most satisfying snack on their own, you might consider topping your salad with them for a little bit of crunch, or pairing them with some berries to make them a little more satisfying.

Probiotics to help boost your gut health.

Probiotics can be found in a number of different ways in health food stores, but they can make digestion and gut health much more optimum. Having a happy gut often means that your dietary success and overall health will improve!

Vegetables that are rich in healthy fats.

Not to sound topical or trendy, but avocados are a great example of a vegetable that is packed with healthy fats. Look for vegetables with fatty acids and a higher fat content and you will find that if you add more of those into your regimen, you will get hungry less often.

Water, water, water, and more water.

No matter what you decide to add to or subtract from your regimen, *stay hydrated.* This will aid in digestive health and ease, it will keep you from feeling as slumpy or tired, and it will keep you from getting too hungry. Add electrolytes where you need to and don't be shy about bringing a bottle with you when you go from place to place. Stay hydrated!

What to Avoid

Any foods that make you feel sad, slow, tired, or gross. Those are the foods to avoid. It's the beginning of a new regimen and it's time for you to stick with foods that make you feel *good!* If you find that a food makes you ill or slows your progress, cut it out!

Macronutrients

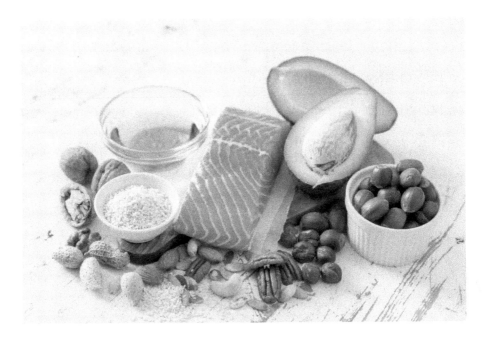

What are Macros?

You have probably heard the term "macronutrients" before, or at least you've heard the term "macros." In many cases, you will hear people on the ketogenic diet talking about them because tracking them is a huge part of that regimen. Tracking your macros should be a huge part of just about any regimen, regardless of it being ketogenic or not.

Macronutrients are, quite simply, the nutritional compounds or elements that you're putting into your body when you eat. The most common ones to watch are protein, carbohydrates, and fats. The reason for looking at these is to make sure that you're keeping things in an adequate balance in your diet. If you're eating mostly fat without eating enough protein or enough carbohydrates, your body will react differently. If you know you need to be eating a certain amount of protein each day, then you will keep a keener eye out for the things that have more of it like chicken breasts, or other lean meats, as they will add protein without adding considerable fat.

In most cases, there aren't rigid numbers you need to stick for each of these while doing intermittent fasting. It is important, however, that you're not taking on foods that are mostly carbs or fat while you're dieting, right? If you want to make sure that your body is going to get the most out of the things you're eating without feeling sluggish or putting on excess weight, you're not going to be eating things that are primarily carbohydrates either.

Carbohydrates

Your body will primarily use carbs as its means of fuel and most typical diets will dictate that you make up your diet with about

45%-65% carbs. Your body will use carbohydrates as the fuel for just about every internal process it has. Your body can very easily break down carbohydrates, making it a convenient fuel source when taken on in the right amounts. There are some doctor-recommended programs for those who need to reduce their weight that require that this percentage be drastically reduced, but that's not typical.

Carbohydrates, when they break down, are converted into glucose, which is the real raw fuel your body can use to keep moving. Glucose is absorbed into the cells of your body, fueling each one's processes. When your body ends up with an excess of glucose, it gets converted once more into something else called glycogen which is converted into the fat stores your body keeps for future use. This is sort of an evolutionary holdover that allows you to get through periods of starvation, as food was far scarcer than it is today. However, most of us are in no position to starve and those fat stores stick around doing no good for anyone until we work them off.

One of the things to bear in mind when you're evaluating whether or not to cut carbohydrates is that there is no one type of carbohydrate and that deciding "carbs are bad," is not as black and white or correct as it might seem. There are simple carbohydrates and there are complex carbohydrates.

The labels "simple" and "complex" refer to the length of the molecule itself, which is obviously not something you'll be able to tell just by looking at the food. You will, however, be able to know it by whether or not the food is processed. Simple carbohydrates that take your body almost no time to burn through and your body will typically be left with more glycogen at the end of that process. Complex carbohydrates take a longer time to break down in the body and give your body more fuel in the time it takes to break them down.

Simple carbohydrates are mostly sugars, so you'll find those in candies, sodas, juices, and things like that. Complex carbohydrates are in things like bananas, legumes, and whole grains.

There is no black and white answer about whether simple or complex carbs are better or worse for you, but you will generally find that complex carbs are much better for *lasting power*. You will, however, find that if you avoid processed foods, you will feel better and get the most out of the carbs that you do eat!

Protein

Proteins are used to build muscle and repair the body to keep it going from day to day. That's why you need more protein if you decide to start working out and exercising more. Your body needs to recuperate and repair and protein is the ideal helper for that process. It's recommended that about 20%-35% of your daily intake is made up of proteins.

The protein that you take on allows your body to restore cells, to grow, to grow your hair and nails, to repair and refresh your skin, and all that very essential stuff! This doesn't mean that eating 100% protein will help your body regenerate like a comic book character, but it does mean that it's quite important to ensure that you're getting enough protein!

You get essential amino acids from the foods that you eat, and those will often come from the animal proteins that you eat. There are 20 amino acids and nine of those aren't produced in our bodies. They're classified as essential because we need to get them from the foods that we eat, namely the animal proteins. If you're a vegetarian, you can get them from sources of plant-based protein.

Fat

Over the decades, you've likely watched the stigma and public opinion surrounding fats evolve. For a while, every diet food was fat-free, then there was the Atkins craze and food couldn't have enough fat in it to satisfy shoppers and dieters, and it's been an ever-evolving cycle ever since. Without getting too confusing about the truth of fats, here is the long and short of it. Fats should take up about 10%-35% of your daily intake. Of those fats, you want to make sure that as many as possible are "good fats."

This means you want fats from lean protein sources, fats that contain Omega-3 fatty acids, Omega-6 fatty acids, and which don't come from overly processed foods. These come from things like fish, walnuts, eggs, and vegetable oils. When foods naturally have fat in them without any help from processes like homogenization or emulsification, you will generally find the fats to be good. The fats in dairy are helpful to the body in moderation, and if you aren't lactose intolerant.

You can also look for these things:

Saturated Fats – These come from meat, dairy, and other animal byproducts.

Unsaturated Fats – These are the plant-based fats that come from veggies, nuts, and the like.

Trans Fats – These types of fats are generally only produced in the commercial production and processing of foods like fast foods, snack foods, and butter substitutes that aren't plant-based.

Trans fats should be avoided for the most part, if not entirely, as those are fats your body can't particularly use and which don't contribute to healthy heart function.

What Should My Macros be During Intermittent Fasting?

There is no set amount of each macro that you should be taking on each day when you're doing intermittent fasting. You will find that you generally want to keep to the percentages outlined above for your macros. That means that you should be eating enough to fill you up without going overboard. In many cases, you will lose weight on intermittent fasting because you won't eat as much as you otherwise would.

Those macros once again are:

Carbs: 45% to 65%
Protein: 20% to 35%
Fats: 10% to 35%

If you are able to make sure your macros are just about in this range, then you will often find that you are feeling your best and that you are doing quite well. If you need the help of a calorie-tracking app, you might find that you're more able to stay on top of your intake and that you're able to feel fuller for longer without overdoing it.

It's not completely necessary to watch your calories in order to do intermittent fasting and to feel the benefits that it has to offer, but it can help you to keep on track and to keep yourself from doing things you wish you hadn't. You might even find that some of your favorite foods are even better for you than you had initially anticipated!

Unfortunately, many of us are not familiar with serving sizes and how much of things we're supposed to be eating in a sitting. Many of us have taken out cues from the restaurants around us and, the horrible truth is that the average restaurant will serve you 2-3 times as much as you're supposed to be eating in one sitting!

If you have found yourself wondering why you're not losing weight when you think you've been eating everything in moderation, it could be worth it to track your calorie and food intake on one of those apps to see what you're really taking in.

Fasting Methods

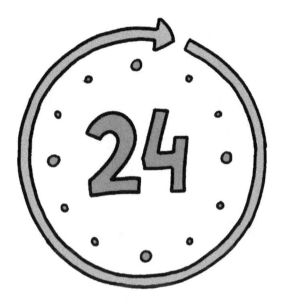

When it comes to choosing the way in which you fast, you aren't forced to choose one method or another. You might find that you're far more able to go without a meal than you thought, or you might find that you're a little bit more dependent on food than you initially anticipated. This is not a problem at all and it should be the basis for your choosing which fasting method works best for you.

Listening to your body is the best way to understand which fasting schedule works best for you and there are no right or wrong answers. The ways in which you will determine which method works best for you is by gauging your weight loss (if that is a goal of yours), your overall health, how you feel, and the quality of your sleep, your metabolism, and your gut health. By watching these things, you will get an accurate picture of whether or not the regimen is working for you.

You will find that the results differ greatly depending on the person and the methods they decide work best for them, so you will want to keep an eye on how you're doing, rather than comparing your own progress with the people around you. If you're feeling like you're not getting the results you feel you should be getting and if you feel like you're not doing as well between meals as you think you should be, then take a look at your regimen and make changes when and where you need to.

You're not committed to your fasting methods throughout the duration of your use of this process. You can make changes when and where it suits you to do so, but make sure that you're picking something that works for you and rolling with it for long enough that your body can adapt, adjust, and get the most out of it.

Some people will try to do intermittent fasting without changing anything about the things that they're eating. Many people who do this will still see some kind of improvements in their lifestyle and their weight, but it is far less than they would see if they improved their intake. It's a great idea to make sure that you're eating nourishing, wholesome foods in between your fasts and that you're not going too overboard on the number of calories you're taking on while considering the calories you're expending in your daily activity and exercise.

You should do your best to keep from binge eating at all while you're doing intermittent fasting, though it's imperative that if you do find yourself eating a lot, that you're not eating lots of junk foods or unhealthy foods. Taking on large quantities of fast foods, junk foods, or unhealthy foods will not yield any health benefits for you and it won't help you to lose weight with any quickness. You must make sure that you're minding your food groups and taking on only what your body can use to keep you going and to improve its functions.

If you find that you have kind of a hard time telling when you've had a full serving of something or more, you may want to start using one of the apps for your smartphone that will tell you what calories and nutrients are in the foods that you're eating. Doing this can give you a more general idea of what a serving of food looks like and how to keep more or less to that region so you're not overeating. This can also give your body the chance to get used to sustaining itself on the right amount of food for a sitting.

While there is not a strict number of calories that you need to stay within during your time doing intermittent fasting, it's important that you're giving your body enough food and nutrition to work with, without overloading it entirely. Weight loss when you're taking on more food than you ought to be will often be more difficult.

The 16/8 Fast

This method dictates that you fast each day of the week for 14-16 hours, leaving yourself only 8 hours to eat. Many people will center this approach right after dinner, and extending it out into the early morning or afternoon. It's a good idea not to eat anything within two to three hours of going to bed for the night so your body has a chance to process all the food you're giving it without keeping you awake.

You will find that most methods don't rely on being overly complex about how and when you eat. Most people who are doing this method will typically just skip their breakfast and eat two meals and some snacks in the latter part of their day, stopping eating at about 8 PM. Let's take a look at how this could look on a calendar.

	Midnight	4 AM	8 AM	12 AM	4 PM	8 PM	Midnight
Day 1	FAST			First meal	Last meal by 8 PM	FAST	
Day 2	FAST			First meal	Last meal by 8 PM	FAST	
Day 3	FAST			First meal	Last meal by 8 PM	FAST	
Day 4	FAST			First meal	Last meal by 8 PM	FAST	
Day 5	FAST			First meal	Last meal by 8 PM	FAST	
Day 6	FAST			First meal	Last meal by 8 PM	FAST	
Day 7	FAST			First meal	Last meal by 8 PM	FAST	

It is not required that you fast every single day when you're doing intermittent fasting, but if it is something that you would like to do daily, this regimen exists to accommodate that preference. This mostly just means that you will be skipping breakfasts and cutting out any nighttime eating.

Nighttime eating can be the reason for a lot of weight gain if you're someone who gets particularly hungry after the sun goes down. Don't worry, you're not alone, but it is a habit you should try your hardest to break. Snacking after dinner can lead to weight gain as you're not particularly active in that part of the day and your body doesn't really have much need for a lot of energy (food) at that time of day.

Skipping breakfast can be very difficult for people who are accustomed to eating in the mornings and some might find that starting their day off by skipping breakfast is a complete deal-breaker. This is also completely fine and you're more than welcome to shift the fast to a different portion of the day so your fast covers dinner instead of breakfast. This will allow you to have more free time in your evenings as well, as you won't need to spend that time cooking anything.

	Midnight	4 AM	8 AM	12 AM	4 PM	8 PM	Midnight
Day 1	FAST	FAST	First meal	Last meal by 4 PM	FAST	FAST	FAST
Day 2	FAST	FAST	First meal	Last meal by 4 PM	FAST	FAST	FAST
Day 3	FAST	FAST	First meal	Last meal by 4 PM	FAST	FAST	FAST
Day 4	FAST	FAST	First meal	Last meal by 4 PM	FAST	FAST	FAST
Day 5	FAST	FAST	First meal	Last meal by 4 PM	FAST	FAST	FAST
Day 6	FAST	FAST	First meal	Last meal by 4 PM	FAST	FAST	FAST
Day 7	FAST	FAST	First meal	Last meal by 4 PM	FAST	FAST	FAST

This would allow you to have your breakfast, your lunch, and some snacks before breaking off for your fast at 4 PM. Your fast would begin right before dinner time, through bedtime, and you would be able to eat within two to three hours or getting your morning started, depending on how early or late your schedule allows you to sleep in.

These are not the only two configurations allowed for this method, of course. If you work third shift or you simply have a different eight-hour window in your day that would make this regimen easier, then, by all means, please commit to that schedule. If you find yourself having trouble sticking to the regimen once you set it, then you may want to take a look at how you can amend, but that's a great place to start!

5:2 Day Cutback

This method is a little bit different in that there aren't two full days of the week during which you don't eat. There are five full days during which you get all of your meals with proper nutrition laid out in a way that is ideal for you and your lifestyle. Two days out of the week, however, you cut your intake down severely. For women, this means that you will be getting about

500 calories per day and you will want to make sure that you're getting protein in those calories and paying special attention to the supplements that you're taking on those days.

If you're unable to take your supplements on these days, you might find that you have a harder time making it through the day. This is because your body is struggling to get all the energy and fuel it needs in order to keep you going and feeling your best. Taking supplements is a very simple fix, however, and adding protein to your day can do wonders for your overall feeling of wellness as well as your state of mind when getting through these two days of your week.

Here is an example calendar for you to follow when you're doing the 5:2 fasting method. As always, there is no reason for you to have to lay your week out in exactly this manner, however, it is *highly* recommended that whatever configuration you settle on, you don't place your two fasting days side by side. It's a wonderful idea to put at *least* one day of normal intake between these two days, as your body will benefit from all the nutrients it will be getting while you're eating normally.

You can see in this diagram that you will have four days in a row of eating normally on days 6, 7, 1, & 2 if you decide to run each of your weeks like this, one right after another. This leaves one day directly in between your fasts.

Day 1	Day 2	Day 3	Day 4	Day 5	Day 6	Day 7
Eat normally	Eat normally	Cut calories down to about 500 per day	Eat normally	Cut calories down to about 500 per day	Eat normally	Eat normally

If you would like a little more balance, you can put two days in between them, you will find your week will look a little more like this:

Day 1	Day 2	Day 3	Day 4	Day 5	Day 6	Day 7
Eat normally	Eat normally	Cut calories down to about 500 per day	Eat normally	Eat normally	Cut calories down to about 500 per day	Eat normally

Even more balanced still would be:

Day 1	Day 2	Day 3	Day 4	Day 5	Day 6	Day 7
Eat normally	Cut calories down to about 500 per day	Eat normally	Eat normally	Eat normally	Cut calories down to about 500 per day	Eat normally

This could be your Monday and Friday (if that works best for you) and then you can eat normally on the weekends and the midweek between those days.

There is truly a method that can fit any schedule and any preference.

5:2 Day Fasting

The diagrams for this method will look fairly familiar to you, as this is simply the method outlined above with fasting instead of cutting down calories. If you have done the 500-calorie days and you have found that you're ready for something a little bit more intensive, this could be a great next step. These arrangements allow you to simply take two days out of your week with no calorie intake at all.

It's imperative, just like with the other methods that you ensure your intake is ideal on the days when you are eating. This will set you up for the best possible success on the days when you're not eating anything at all.

Even if you preceded this regimen with a routine of eating 500 calories on those days of the week, you might find it to be difficult to get through the full-day fasts in the very beginning. It's important to give yourself time to adjust to those periods and to expect that you may not be operating at peak levels during those times.

Consider upping the amount of protein you're taking on in the days when you eat normally and consider upping the quality of carbohydrates that you're taking in on the days on either side of your fasts. By doing this, your body will have more nutrients to work with and you'll be filling in any gaps caused by the lack of nutrition on those days.

Day 1	Day 2	Day 3	Day 4	Day 5	Day 6	Day 7
Eat normally	Eat normally	24-hour fast	Eat normally	24-hour fast	Eat normally	Eat normally

If you would like a little more balance, you can put two days in between them, you will find your week will look a little more like this:

Day 1	Day 2	Day 3	Day 4	Day 5	Day 6	Day 7
Eat normally	Eat normally	24-hour fast	Eat normally	Eat normally	24-hour fast	Eat normally

Even more balanced still would be:

Day 1	Day 2	Day 3	Day 4	Day 5	Day 6	Day 7
Eat normally	24-hour fast	Eat normally	Eat normally	Eat normally	24-hour fast	Eat normally

This could be your Monday and Friday (if that works best for you) and then you can eat normally on the weekends and the midweek between those days.

3:4 Day Cutback

Just as you may be able to deduce from the name of this method, this is very similar to the 5:2 Day Cutback, only you've added a whole extra day to your week with a lowered calorie intake. This would once again be that 500-calorie limit, but you can and should make amendments to this method as your body needs you to do so.

It's important to make sure, as always, that you're watching your nutrients and that you're getting enough of everything on the days when you're not fasting, without overdoing it. This might require a gradual approach so you can get a feel for the way your body handles schedules like this.

Day 1	Day 2	Day 3	Day 4	Day 5	Day 6	Day 7
Eat normally	Cut calories down to about 500 per day	Eat normally	Cut calories down to about 500 per day	Eat normally	Cut calories down to about 500 per day	Eat normally

When you're doing this method, this is more or less the best way to do it. You will have two days between two of your fasts and one day between the others.

As with the 5:2, you don't want to put any two 500-calorie days right next to each other if you can avoid it. If you do find this is something you would like to work toward anyway, you might consider not starting off that way. You might want to consider working up to that method.

You can cut your meals down to 250 calories each, or you can break them up further and do little snacks in between, but it's important these are as nutrient-rich as possible. Don't forget your supplements! I know I sound like a broken record about the supplements, but you won't believe the difference they'll make until you miss out on them!

3:4 Day Fasting

This method is even more hardcore than the last, as it requires that you fast three days out of the week with a minimum of one day in between fasts.

Day 1	Day 2	Day 3	Day 4	Day 5	Day 6	Day 7
Eat normally	24-hour fast	Eat normally	24-hour fast	Eat normally	24-hour fast	Eat normally

It is recommended that on this method, you get as much nutrition into those other four days as possible and that you continue to take your supplements on the off days in any way you can. If your supplements cannot be taken on an empty stomach, consider having one yogurt in the mornings so you can take them, but abstaining from food for the rest of the day. Again, your doctor may have more sound advice on this method, but that's a great place to start!

The Warrior Diet

This is the method that a lot of people find works best for them, as it allows them to eat something each day while still providing benefits. The long and short of this method is that you will eat nothing until around dinnertime, then have one large meal to tide you over throughout your next (immediate) fast.

This does seem like it goes against the idea of avoiding binging or large meals in between fasts, but since they're the *only* meal your body will be taking on over an extended period of time, your body can and will store that food and disburse those nutrients over the course of the next 24 hours.

Most people like to give themselves about a four-hour window during which they can take on their food for the day, as it eliminates the need for a rush to get in all the calories that will get them through their next fast.

So if you like to do The Warrior diet, you can arrange it around whatever meal works best for you.

Eating breakfast:

	Day 1	Day 2	Day 3	Day 4	Day 5	Day 6	Day 7
Midnight / 4 AM	FAST	FAST	FAST	FAST	FAST	FAST	FAST
8 AM	Eat	Eat	Eat	Eat	Eat	Eat	Eat
12 AM							
4 PM / 8 PM / Midnight	FAST	FAST	FAST	FAST	FAST	FAST	FAST

Eating lunch:

	Midnight	4 AM	8 AM	12 AM	4 PM	8 PM	Midnight
Day 1	FAST	FAST		Eat		FAST	FAST
Day 2	FAST	FAST		Eat		FAST	FAST
Day 3	FAST	FAST		Eat		FAST	FAST
Day 4	FAST	FAST		Eat		FAST	FAST
Day 5	FAST	FAST		Eat		FAST	FAST
Day 6	FAST	FAST		Eat		FAST	FAST
Day 7	FAST	FAST		Eat		FAST	FAST

Eating dinner:

	Midnight	8 PM	4 PM	12 AM	8 AM	4 AM	Midnight
Day 1	FAST		Eat			FAST	
Day 2	FAST		Eat			FAST	
Day 3	FAST		Eat			FAST	
Day 4	FAST		Eat			FAST	
Day 5	FAST		Eat			FAST	
Day 6	FAST		Eat			FAST	
Day 7	FAST		Eat			FAST	

It should work well to align your supplements with your dinner, so long as nothing you're taking will interrupt your sleep patterns!

Tips & Tricks for Effective Weight Loss with Intermittent Fasting

As hard as it might be, do not binge between fasts. Your body will only get hungrier later on. A controlled intake is best.

You might find that, as soon as you come off of a fast, you're running right to the refrigerator and eating just about anything you can get your hands on. This is completely normal, but it can actually set you back. It's a great idea to have something made by the time your fast ends, so you can reach for it and dig in. However, you will want to make sure that you're having a regular-sized portion of food and that you give it a little bit of time to settle before reaching for something more, like snacks.

Conversely, make sure that you don't start your fasts right after a huge meal. You'll start off feeling much more ready to face your fast, but your hunger will come back much more quickly and with a vengeance! In order to keep those fierce hunger pangs at bay, have normally-sized portions at regular intervals between fasts.

97

Consult with your doctor about the ideal supplements for you while you're fasting and take them regularly.

When you're cutting some foods out of your regimen, your body misses out on some of the opportunities it has to get the nutrients it needs in order to run strong. Speak with your doctor about what supplements are ideal for you and consider adding them into your daily regimen.

While it's ideal to take your supplements in the morning for most people, it can hurt your stomach to take them when you're fasting. Speak with your doctor about the best time of day to take your supplements with food so you get the maximum benefit from them without interrupting your sleep cycle. Certain vitamins like B-complex can wake you up shortly after you take them, making them a poor choice for bedtime consumption.

Don't get too caught up in the nitty-gritty details of how your fasts should be structured; pick something that works for you and roll with it.

It can be easy to get overwhelmed by all the information and all the options when you first introduce yourself to the subject of intermittent fasting. It's important to remember that you don't need to commit everything to memory before you get started. Simply look at the options that are available to you, pick the one that looks most beneficial or doable to you, and get started with that. Once you're on a regimen, you can adapt as you need to and you can always learn more as you continue on with this process.

Don't over-exert yourself when exercising.

You will find that if you push yourself really hard when you're working out, you will need a lot of recovery time and more food to help your body bounce back from that exertion. You can absolutely exercise while you're doing intermittent fasting, but it's important (especially in the beginning) not to overdo it while you're fasting or even between fasts so you're not giving your system too much to deal with on the amount of nutrients that you're taking on. Some trial and error might be needed in order to find a balance that works for you. If you find it difficult to find that balance, consult with your doctor for recommendations on how to move forward.

Drink plenty of water.

Staying hydrated is an essential part of life in general and should be kept in mind whenever you're doing any dietary regimen. When you're fasting, however, you will find that keeping yourself hydrated can assist your metabolism in the adjustments that it needs to make, and that it can contribute to your feeling of overall wellness.

If you find that you're drinking lots of water and that you're not really getting any benefit from it, or you're just constantly going to the bathroom without finding any sort of difference, you might want to incorporate electrolytes into your daily intake so your body can more easily use the water that you're giving your system.

Ensure that you're eating whole, nourishing foods in between fasts.

There are some sources that will tell you that, so long as you're doing intermittent fasting, you won't need to make any changes to the foods you're eating in order to get a benefit from it. This isn't the approach this book recommends that you take, but you may find that suggestion in your travels and in your research.

It is recommended that the food you eat between fasts is healthy, nourishing, and satisfying for you so that you can get the absolute most out of your regimen. You will find that the recipes in this book are not particularly focused on cutting out certain things like fat carbs, or natural sugars, but that they do take things in moderation.

There are some meals that are particularly carb-y and you're more than welcome to cut those down if you feel most comfortable with that, but the idea is to take on the right nutrients in between your fasts so your body has the best, cleanest fuel possible to keep yourself going and to optimize while fasting! You may also find that if you stick to these recipes and eat only foods that contain the best whole ingredients, that you simply feel better and more satisfied.

Get plenty of rest, especially after a workout.

Your body needs sleep on a consistent basis and you will often find that you feel better when you concentrate on consistently getting enough rest. If you're working out or exercising frequently, it's imperative to ensure that you're getting good sleep that night. Your body will recuperate much more quickly and you'll feel much better after a while.

Give it 30 days to see if you really like intermittent fasting.

Intermittent fasting, like any other regimen, simply isn't for everyone. You might find that, even after a whole month, it's not for you. That's perfectly okay and there might just be a better regimen out there for you somewhere. You may find, though, that your body simply needs to take advantage of an adjustment period to get used to everything that comes with intermittent fasting. Give yourself one month or 30 days to adjust to everything that you're supposed to do while fasting and do your best to stick to your routine in that time. Your body may need a little time to catch on, so take that 30 days and see how you feel!

If you find that your hunger is intense during fasts, try cutting carbs

You might start to feel like your hunger is getting the best of you when you're fasting and that you simply can't make it that long between meals. This isn't abnormal when you're starting out, but if it persists, you might find that you need to cut down the amount of carbs you're taking on when you're between fasts. Excess carbs can burn off more quickly than you might expect and you might find and they can actually make you hungrier much sooner than you otherwise might be. You can cut back on carbs and slightly kick up your protein and fiber to see if that helps things.

If you're feeling ill, put the fasting on hold.

Illness happens. Sometimes we get blindsided with a stomach bug or a head cold and it's imperative that we exercise proper health and nutrition during those times. Starving a fever has proven to make them last longer, so it's best to keep your body fed and rested so it can fight off whatever bugs might be attacking your system. This doesn't mean you should be eating lots of the wrong foods, though. Your body needs high-quality nutrients in order to fuel it against the illness in your body, so be kind and eat the right things.

Keep an eye on how you feel at all times, and if you feel like you're not doing well with intermittent fasting, stop and consult your doctor.

We all have off-days when we're not feeling our best, but if you find that you're consistently feeling hungry, tired, stressed, run-down, or other negative feelings, then you might want to make some adjustments to your regimen. If you're not sure how to proceed or what to change in order to make sure your body is supported, consult with your doctor and see if they have suggestions about how best to proceed and support your health.

Keep yourself busy and find things to occupy your time in between meals.

A lot of us struggle with the impulse to eat when we're bored. A lot of us also struggle to forget that we've gone a long stretch in between our meals when we're not otherwise engaged or occupied. If you find yourself with a lot of downtime while you're fasting, consider picking up a hobby or other activity that keeps your mind engaged and which keeps you committed to tasks. This can help you to keep your mind on other things and it can even keep the hunger response from kicking in from time to time.

Make sure the meals that you're eating are satisfying.

While you don't want to have meals that are overly large between your fasts, you also want to make sure that they're not too scant. You will want to make sure that the meals you're preparing for yourself are nutritious and satisfying so you're well-fed and provided with the best possible nourishment to carry you through your fasts. It may take a few attempts before you feel like your meals will carry you through, but keeping your nutrients balanced and ensuring that you're getting the right amount of protein should help you adjust very well.

Make sure you're getting enough protein to compensate for the times when you're not eating.

As above, you will want to make sure that you're eating enough protein. Protein is a nutrient that has a lot of sticking power and which can hold you over for a longer period of time. Combining carbohydrates and protein in the right measures can go a long way to keep you satisfied until your next meal. Hardboiled eggs make a great snack that are mostly protein and fat. Combined with a little bit of something with carbohydrates, it's a snack that can carry you through a few hours quite easily!

Manage your expectations and don't take setbacks too hard.

Intermittent fasting and its benefits are not achieved easily and on the first day. These are things that are achieved over time and with dedication. You may find that you can't get through your first fast without having a little bit of something to tide you over. That is completely fine and you don't need to beat yourself up over something like that. You will find that, as you continue on with the regimen, it will get easier and easier to acclimate yourself to the process, and you will find that you feel better and better as you continue to try at it. You may even need to scale back your fasts in the beginning and lengthen them little by little over time. This is also completely fine as long as you're feeling better and doing well. That is the number one goal.

Once you form a routine, do your best to stick to it. Your body thrives on regularity.

Once you have found your fasting "sweet spot," and you know you can stick to that without too much difficulty, it's a great idea to support that regimen for a sustained period of time. This means that you will want to keep special occasions from interjecting into the middle of your routine, this means you won't want to add new things to what you're eating for a little while, and it means that you'll want to keep your fasting routine stable. Life happens and there are always exceptions, but when you're doing your best to keep your routine supported, you will often feel your best.

Pay attention to what your body is telling you and consult with your doctor whenever necessary.

If you are feeling things that indicate that something is wrong, or if you're feeling unwell, you must listen to your body. Don't push through the things that could be indicators of an illness. Do your best to differentiate between the growing pains of a new regimen and indications that your body is unwell. If you feel like you're malnourished, like you're faint or dizzy, or like there may be something wrong, stay in communication with your doctor to ensure that you're getting everything that your body needs. You don't want to deprive your body of the supplements and nutrients that it needs in order to survive!

Practice mindfulness so you can be more aware of how you're feeling from day to day and make necessary changes.

Mindfulness exercises have been used to help people to lessen stress in their lives, but many have also found that when they practice mindfulness, they simply become more aware of their surroundings and of themselves. Many have found that by practicing mindfulness, they weren't so preoccupied with life and all the things going on around them to be able to tell when something shifted and they weren't doing as well as they had been doing before.

Staying acutely aware of how your body is responding to regimen changes can really help you to stay ahead of the curve and to eliminate routines and behaviors that don't contribute to a healthier, happier, and better lifestyle for you.

Speak with your doctor about whether you could benefit from a regimen of Branch Chain Amino Acids (BCAAs).

BCAAs are often used in order to combat fatigue and muscle soreness. If you're finding that it's hard for you to get the rest and recovery you need after workouts, it could mean that you need to add this supplement to your regimen in order to help you move on from those workouts and to get the maximum benefits of them.

Start off with a shorter fasting period.

In the very beginning, you may want to start with the shorter fast. You can acclimate to the fast over time and extend it as you get more used to doing things on this system. It's always best to work up to something harder than to over-extend yourself the first time around and give yourself a bad experience right at the very beginning.

If you try to go too long between meals in the very beginning, you could experience a number of unpleasant things like nausea, feeling faint, hunger pangs, nausea, mood swings, and some other things. It can be really hard to convince yourself it's worth it to keep trying when you're forcing yourself to go through those symptoms a couple of times.

Starting off with a shorter fast allows you more time to get accustomed to how things work and then encourages you to increase the length of your fast over time.

Take regular walks.

Walking is wonderful for your health and it can do wonders for your mental health as well. Gain a little bit of clarity of mind, get your blood pumping, take in the scenery, and don't overdo it. Just a light walk a couple of times a day can improve your digestion, your blood flow, the way your muscles feel, and it can help you to keep your mind off of the hunger you may be feeling as well if you're keeping yourself occupied.

Take up something relaxing like meditation.

Keeping your stress level low is a great way to encourage better health and to keep you from feeling like you're snowed under when you're experiencing a lot of changes. If meditation is something that works for you, then you might find the regular practice of it to be a great benefit to you while you're getting used to how things work. There are many wonderful resources to assist you in learning how to meditate and get the most out of it. Feel free to look into those and adopt meditation into your regimen.

Try to start your fasts after dinner so you're asleep for a good portion of your fast.

It's possible to line up your fasts to begin right after dinner so you're sleeping for about 8 hours of your fasting time. In such cases, it's a good idea to extend your fast so it does take over the slot of time during which you would typically be having your breakfast. Otherwise, it's not much of a change, is it?

This is a little leg-up helper that can make getting acclimated less difficult for you and it's something that you might want to try if you find yourself struggling to fast.

Use coffee or tea to tide you over between meals and to occupy your palate between meals.

While no one is recommending that you drastically increase your coffee or caffeine intake (especially if it goes against what your doctor instructs you to do), it can be helpful to have something to ingest during fasts like coffee, tea, herbal tea, sparkling water, or flavored waters (preferably flavored with essence with no artificial sweeteners) to help occupy your palate. This can often make it easier to make it to your next meal, as it breaks up the monotony of not tasting anything between meals. It might be hard to consider, but it may surprise you what an impact this has in the very beginning.

When you feel a wave of hunger, try to ride it out. Distraction helps.

It's possible to feel pangs of hunger in between meals. When this happens, try to do something to keep your mind occupied and to keep you from thinking too much about the fact that you're hungry. It's typical for that hunger response to shut itself down if your body realizes that there's no food coming at the moment and that it will need to figure out how to wait it out.

Breakfast Recipes

Sweet Potato Hash

Number of Servings: 4 | Prep Time: 10 min. | Cook Time: 30 min.

Calories: 390 | Carbohydrates: 44g | Fat: 16g | Protein: 17g | Sugar: 14g

Ingredients:

½ tsp. cumin

½ tsp. salt

1 lg. bell pepper, diced

1 med. onion, diced

1 tsp. garlic powder

1.5 lb. sweet potatoes, cubed

2 c. frozen spinach, chopped, thawed, & drained

2 med. green onions, sliced

2 tbsp. avocado oil (or oil of preference)

4 lg. eggs

6 oz. turkey sausage, halved & sliced

Ground black pepper, to taste

Red pepper flakes, to taste

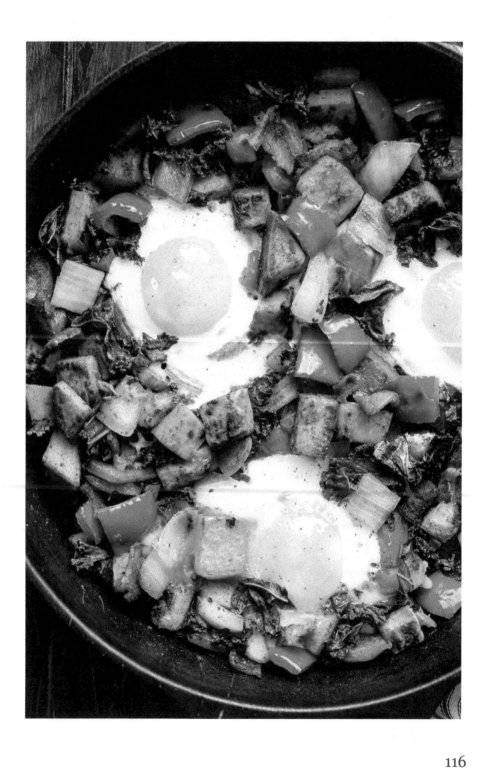

Instructions:

1. Heat a large skillet over medium-high heat and warm the oil in the pan, spreading it evenly over the bottom of the pan.

2. Stir the onion and bell peppers into the pan and heat through until shiny and fragrant, about three minutes.

3. Stir the sausage into the pan along with the garlic powder, sweet potatoes, cumin, pepper flakes, ground pepper, and salt.

4. Stir all ingredients to fully incorporate, then cover the skillet and allow to cook on low heat for 12-15 minutes, stirring a few times throughout. The potatoes should be firm, but cooked.

5. Stir the spinach into the pan until completely incorporated.

6. Using your spoon or spatula, make four little divots or wells into the mixture and crack one egg into each well. Season to taste then cover and allow to cook for another

five minutes or so until the eggs have reached the desired level of doneness.

7. Garnish with green onion and serve hot!

Blueberry Smoothie

Number of Servings: 1 | Prep Time: 5 min. | Cook Time: 0 min.

Calories: 442 | Carbohydrates: 62g | Fat: 13g | Protein: 29g | Sugar: 16g

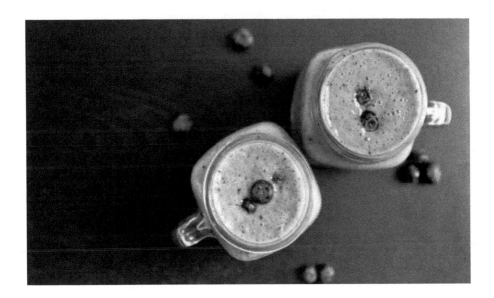

Ingredients:

½ c. quick oats

1 ½ c. almond milk, unsweetened

1 c. blueberries, fresh or frozen

1 scoop nutritional shake powder

Instructions:

1. Combine all ingredients into a blender and blend until completely smooth, scraping down the sides of the jar as needed.

2. Serve cold!

Almond Smoothie

Number of Servings: 1 | Prep Time: 5 min. | Cook Time: 0 min.

Calories: 453 | Carbohydrates: 30g | Fat: 24g | Protein: 31g |

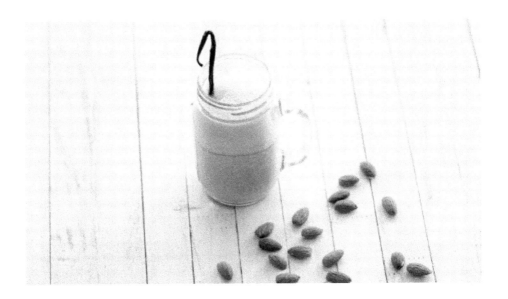

Sugar: 4g

Ingredients:

¼ c. almonds, raw & unsalted

½ c. quick oats

½ tsp. almond extract

1 ¼ c. almond milk, unsweetened

2 scoops vanilla protein powder

Instructions:

1. Combine all ingredients into a blender and blend until completely smooth, scraping down the sides of the jar as needed.

2. Serve chilled!

Bakeless Peanut Butter Bars

Number of Servings: 16 | Prep Time: 30 min. | Chill Time: 30 min.

Calories: 220 | Carbohydrates: 17g | Fat: 15g | Protein: 7g | Sugar: 7g

Ingredients:

¼ c. chocolate chips

¼ c. maple syrup or honey

¼ tsp. salt

½ c. coconut flakes, unsweetened

½ tsp. cinnamon

½ tsp. vanilla extract

1 ½ c. quick oats

1 c. almonds, raw & unsalted

1 c. creamy peanut butter

Instructions:

1. In a food processor, add almonds and allow to process on high until the almonds are ground finely.

2. Combine the oats into the processor and continue until fine and well incorporated.

3. Combine the coconut flakes, salt, cinnamon, and vanilla. Process until well incorporated.

4. Combine the peanut butter and sweetening syrup and process once again until thoroughly combined. Stop to scrape mixture off the sides of the processor periodically, if needed.

5. Add chocolate chips and pulse until well incorporated.

6. Line an 8" x 8" baking dish with wax or parchment paper and pour the dough into the dish. Using your hands and/or your spatula, press the mixture until it's in one even layer in the bottom of the baking dish.

7. Freeze the dish for 30 minutes or until the dough is firm, then slice into 16 evenly-sized squares.

8. Serve!

TIP: Can be stored in an airtight container in the refrigerator for future enjoyment!

High Protein Waffles

Number of Servings: 5 | Prep Time: 3 min. | Cook Time: 30 min.

Calories: 222 | Carbohydrates: 21g | Fat: 8g | Protein: 17g | Sugar: 2g

Ingredients:

¼ c. milk of your choice

2/3 c. Greek yogurt, plain

1 c. oat flour

2 scoops vanilla protein powder

4 lg. eggs

Instructions:

1. Get your waffle iron warming up and combine eggs, yogurt, and milk in a large mixing bowl with a whisk.

2. Add the oat flour and protein powder, whisk until a smooth batter is formed.

3. Using a ¼ cup measure, scoop the batter into the waffle maker and cook per the instructions for the maker.

4. Serve two waffles and enjoy!

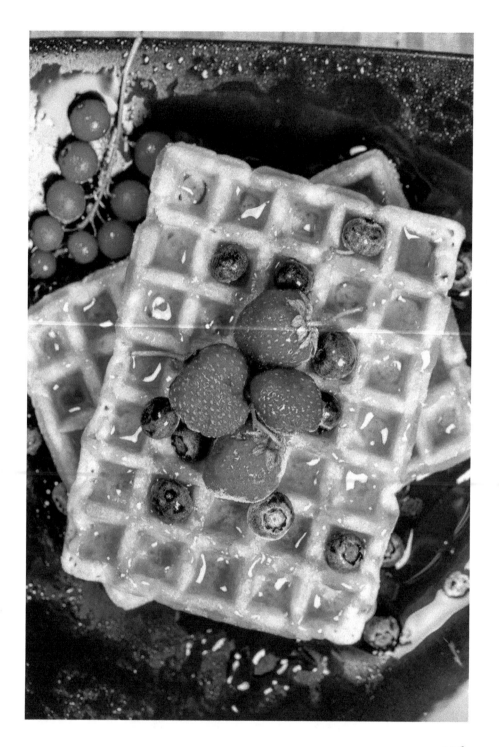

Wholesome Breakfast Bowls

Number of Servings: 4 | Prep Time: 5 min. | Cook Time: 15 min.

Calories: 407 | Carbohydrates: 34g | Fat: 21g | Protein: 25g | Sugar: 9g

Ingredients:

¼ c. water

1 c. cauliflower, chopped

1 tsp. garlic powder

2 c. broccoli, chopped

2 med. bell peppers, diced

2 oz. cheddar cheese, shredded

2 tbsp. avocado oil (or oil of preference)

2 tbsp. salsa

8 lg. eggs

Sea salt & pepper, to taste

Instructions:

1. Heat a large skillet over medium heat and warm your oil in it.

2. Add chopped broccoli and cauliflower to the pan, stir, cover, and allow to cook for two to three minutes. Stir, cover once more, and allow to cook for another two to three minutes.

3. In a small bowl, whisk salt, pepper, eggs, and water until thoroughly combined.

4. Add peppers and garlic powder, adding salt and pepper, to taste once more. Add eggs and stir thoroughly and allow to cook until the eggs are firm, stirring as needed.

5. Divide between 4 airtight containers and store for later use or serve hot!

Grab 'n' Go Egg Muffins

Number of Servings: 12 | Prep Time: 10 min. | Cook Time: 20 min.

Calories: 71 | Carbohydrates: 6g | Fat: 2g | Protein: 8g | Sugar: 1g

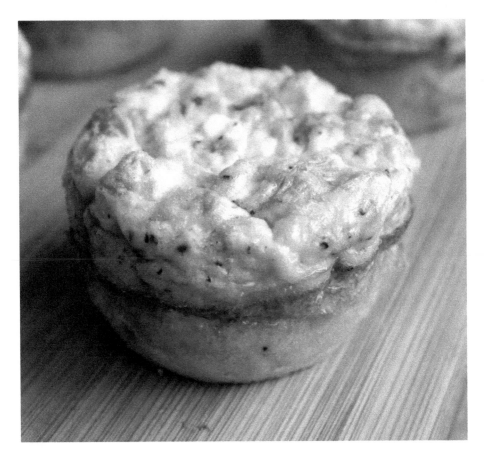

Ingredients:

$1/8$ tsp. red pepper flakes

¼ c. feta cheese crumbles

¼ c. Monterey jack cheese, shredded

½ c. parsley

1 tbsp. onion powder

2 c. broccoli, finely chopped

2 med. green onions, sliced

9 lg. eggs

Non-stick cooking spray (or preferred oil)

Sea salt & pepper, to taste

Instructions:

1. Preheat oven to 350° Fahrenheit and lightly grease your muffin tin with non-stick spray or preferred oil.

2. In a large mixing bowl, beat eggs, then add feta, Monterey jack, onion powder, salt, pepper, pepper flakes, broccoli, parsley, and green onions until thoroughly combined.

3. Pour about ¼ cup of the egg and veggie mixture into each well in the muffin tin until each one is about ¾ of the way full.

4. You can sprinkle a little extra cheese on top if you prefer.

5. Bake for about 20 minutes or until firm all the way through.

6. Allow to cool for about five to ten minutes before removing the eggs from the tin, then serve.

TIP: These can be stored in an airtight container for up to one week, so they're perfect for on-the-go breakfasts!

Creamy Overnight Oats

Number of Servings: 1 | Prep Time: 5 min. | Chill Time: 8 hr.

Calories: 253 | Carbohydrates: 45g | Fat: <1g | Protein: 11g |

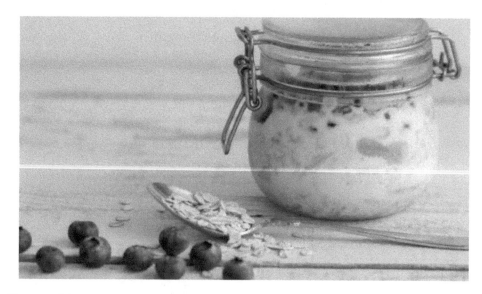

Sugar: 18g

Ingredients:

½ c. quick oats

½ tsp. vanilla extract

¾ c. milk of choice

2 tsp. maple syrup or honey

Instructions:

1. In a medium bowl, combine all ingredients and mix thoroughly until all the ingredients have been fully incorporated.

2. Place the oat mixture into an airtight glass container and move to the refrigerator to chill overnight.

3. Serve topped with berries, banana slices, coconut flakes, or any other topping that you prefer!

TIP: If the mix is just a little bit too thick for you, add a little milk and stir!

Quinoa Granola

Number of Servings: 12 | Prep Time: 5 min. | Cook Time: 30 min.

Calories: 160 | Carbohydrates: 16g | Fat: 9g | Protein: 4g | Sugar: 3g

Ingredients:

1/8 tsp. sea salt

¼ c. chia seeds

¼ c. coconut flakes, unsweetened

½ c. nuts (we used cashews), coarsely chopped

½ c. quinoa, uncooked

1 c. quick oats

1 tsp. vanilla extract

3 tbsp. coconut oil (or preferred oil)

3 tbsp. honey

Instructions:

1. Preheat oven to 325° Fahrenheit and line a baking sheet with parchment paper.

2. In a medium mixing bowl, combine all ingredients except for coconut. Mix well until completely combined.

3. Spread the mixture into one even layer on the baking sheet and bake for 25 minutes.

4. Sprinkle the coconut on top of the granola and return to oven for five more minutes.

5. Let the granola cool completely, then break it up into pieces with your spatula.

6. Transfer the granola to an airtight glass container and store in a cool, dry place for as long as one month.

Lunch Recipes

Beef & Barley Soup

Number of Servings: 8 | Prep Time: 10 min. | Cook Time: 50 min.

Calories: 189 | Carbohydrates: 22g | Fat: 4g | Protein: 16g | Sugar: 3g

Ingredients:

½ c. parsley, finely chopped

½ tsp. thyme, dried

1 c. wheat barley, hulled

1 lb. ground beef

1 lg. onion, diced

1 tbsp. extra virgin olive oil

1 tsp. salt

2 lg. stalks celery, diced

3 bay leaves

3 cloves garlic, minced

3 lg. carrots, diced

9 c. low-sodium beef broth

Ground black pepper, to taste

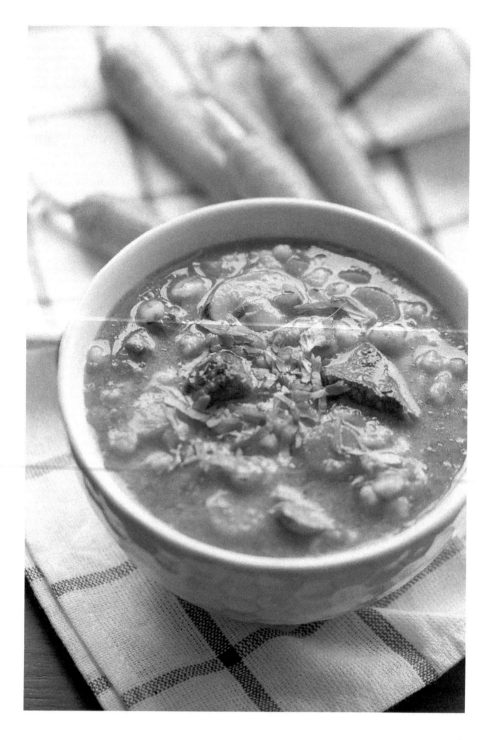

Instructions:

1. Heat a large pot or Dutch oven over medium heat and add oil to it.

2. Once the oil is hot, stir the onion and garlic in, allowing them to cook for about three minutes, stirring often.

3. Stir carrots, beef, celery, and thyme into the pot. Brown the beef, breaking it into smaller chunks as you do so.

4. Once the beef is browned, add the broth, salt, pepper, and bay leaves to the pot, stirring completely. Cover the pot and bring to a boil.

5. Once boiling, reduce the heat to low and let simmer for 40 minutes.

6. Remove the pot from the heat and stir, adding the parsley and adjusting the seasoning to suit your taste. Remove the bay leaves and stir once more.

7. Serve hot!

Instant Pot Chicken

Number of Servings: 6 | Prep Time: 5 min. | Cook Time: 20 min.

Calories: 223 | Carbohydrates: 0g | Fat: 11g | Protein: 30g | Sugar: 0g

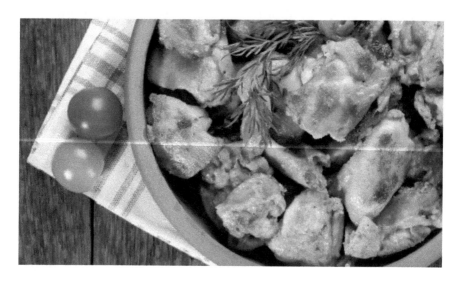

Ingredients:

1 c. water

1 tsp. rosemary, chopped

1 med. lemon, sliced

2 cloves garlic, minced

2 lb. chicken thighs, boneless & skinless

2 tbsp. extra virgin olive oil

Sea salt & pepper, to taste

Instructions:

1. Combine all ingredients in a medium mixing bowl, incorporate fully and cover.

2. Plug in your Instant Pot and select the Sauté setting. Drizzle a little extra olive oil into the bottom of it to prevent sticking.

3. Once the pot is hot, place the thighs in one even layer on the bottom of the Instant Pot and allow to cook until a golden crust is formed on the chick (about four to five minutes, then flip and allow the other side to cook as well.

4. Pull the thighs out of the pot and use the water to deglaze the bottom of the pot, scraping lightly with your spatula or spoon as you stir the water around the pot.

5. Place the chicken into the pot (on top of the trivet insert if you have one, but no problem if you don't) and place the lid on top. Cook at high pressure for five minutes to cook the chicken the rest of the way through.

6. Release the pressure and remove the chicken from the pot.

7. Serve hot with your favorite sides!

Shrimp Salad

Number of Servings: 8 | Prep Time: 15 min. | Cook Time: 0 min.

Calories: 112 | Carbohydrates: 4g | Fat: 5g | Protein: 14g | Sugar: 3g

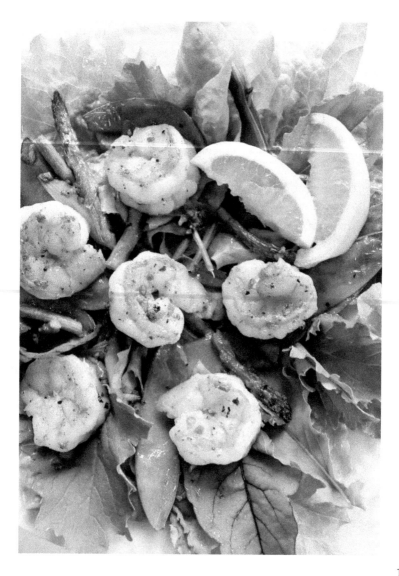

Ingredients:

1/3 English cucumber, diced

¾ c. plain yogurt

1 lb. shrimp, cooked & chopped

1 tbsp. Dijon mustard

1 tsp. garlic powder

2 tbsp. mayo

3 med. stalks celery, diced

Sea salt & pepper, to taste

Instructions:

1. In a large mixing bowl, combine all ingredients and stir to combine thoroughly.

2. Cover and chill for at least 15 minutes before serving.

3. Serve chilled!

Broccoli Salad

Number of Servings: 6 | Prep Time: 20 min. | Cook Time: 5 min.

Calories: 234 | Carbohydrates: 20g | Fat: 13g | Protein: 9g | Sugar: 9g

Ingredients:

½ c. dried cranberries, unsweetened

½ c. pecans, chopped

½ c. sunflower seeds

1 ½ tbsp. onion powder

1 c. plain yogurt

1 lb. broccoli, chopped

1 sm. bell pepper, diced

1 tbsp. apple cider vinegar

Red pepper flakes, to taste

Sea salt & pepper, to taste

Instructions:

1. In a large mixing bowl, combine all ingredients and stir to combine thoroughly.

2. Cover and chill for at least 15 minutes before serving.

3. Serve chilled!

Southwest Chicken Salad

Number of Servings: 8 | Prep Time: 15 min. | Cook Time: 15 min.

Calories: 217 | Carbohydrates: 30g | Fat: 9g | Protein: 7g | Sugar: 2g

Ingredients:

¼ c. extra virgin olive oil

¼ c. red onion, finely chopped

1 c. corn, drained

1 can low-sodium black beans, rinsed & drained

1 jalapeño, seeded & minced

1 tsp. chili powder

1 tsp. cumin

1 tsp. garlic powder

1 tsp. onion powder

2 bell peppers, diced

2 lg. limes, juiced

2 lb. chicken thighs, cooked and diced

2 tbsp. cilantro, finely chopped

3 c. quinoa, cooked to package instructions (still hot)

Sea salt & black pepper, to taste

Instructions:

1. In a small bowl, combine lime juice, chili powder, onion powder, garlic powder, cumin, and cilantro. Mix thoroughly and set aside.

2. In a large mixing bowl, combine all other ingredients and toss until thoroughly combined.

3. Drizzle seasoning mixture over the salad and toss to coat completely.

4. Cover and chill for at least 30 minutes.

5. Serve chilled!

Tuna Salad

Number of Servings: 10 | Prep Time: 15 min. | Cook Time: 0 min.

Calories: 152 | Carbohydrates: 2g | Fat: 8g | Protein: 18g | Sugar: 1g

Ingredients:

¼ c. mayonnaise

¼ c. red onion, finely diced

¾ c. plain yogurt

1 clove garlic, minced

1 lg. stalk celery, diced

1 tbsp. lemon juice

2 sm. dill pickles, diced

24 oz. tuna packed in water, drained

Sea salt & pepper, to taste

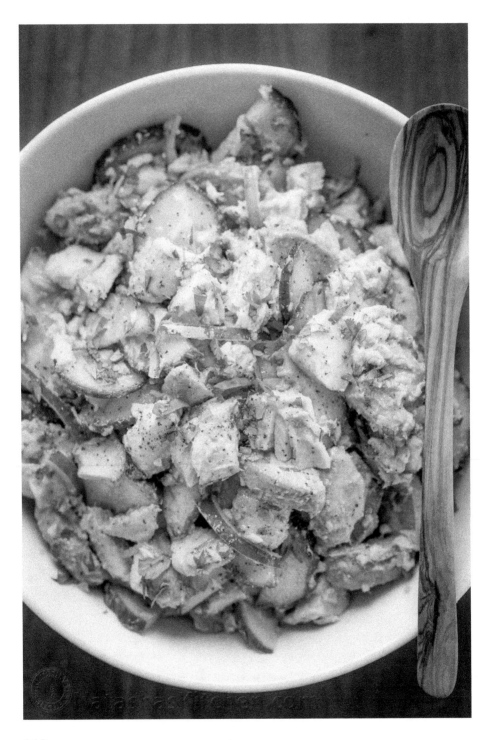

Instructions:

1. In a large mixing bowl, combine all ingredients and stir to combine thoroughly.

2. Cover and chill for at least 15 minutes before serving.

3. Serve chilled!

Black Bean & Quinoa Salad

Number of Servings: 4 | Prep Time: 15 min. | Cook Time: 15 min.

Calories: 408 | Carbohydrates: 53g | Fat: 17g | Protein: 14g |
Sugar: 4g

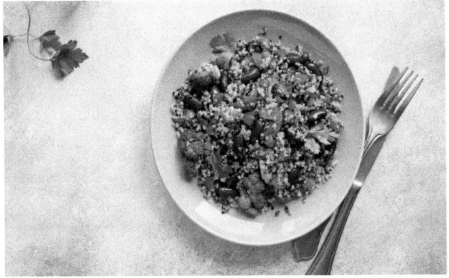

Ingredients:

3 c. quinoa, cooked to package instructions and cooled

14 oz. low-sodium black beans, rinsed and drained

1 lg. tomatoes, diced

2 tbsp. cilantro, finely chopped

¼ c. red onion, finely diced

1 jalapeño, seeded & minced

1 clove garlic, minced

2 lg. limes, juiced

¼ c. extra virgin olive oil

1 tsp. cumin

1 tsp. chili powder

1 tsp. onion powder

Sea salt & pepper to taste

Instructions:

1. In a small bowl, combine olive oil, lime juice, cumin, cilantro, salt, pepper, chili powder, and onion powder. Mix thoroughly.

2. In a large mixing bowl, combine all remaining ingredients and stir to combine thoroughly.

3. Drizzle dressing over the mixture and stir once more to combine.

4. Cover and chill for at least 15 minutes before serving.

5. Serve chilled!

Pasta Salad

Number of Servings: 8 | Prep Time: 8 min. | Cook Time: 10 min.

Calories: 247 | Carbohydrates: 26g | Fat: 15g | Protein: 7g | Sugar: 3g

Ingredients:

$1/8$ tsp. red pepper flakes

$1/3$ c. extra virgin olive oil

$1/3$ c. parsley, finely chopped

½ c. feta cheese crumbles

1 c. Kalamata olives pitted and halved

1 lb. fresh green beans, chopped

1 tbsp. oregano

2 tsp. garlic powder

4 sm. tomatoes, diced

8 oz. whole-grain macaroni, cooked al dente and cooled

Sea salt & pepper to taste

Instructions:

1. Place chopped green beans into a small pot of water and heat over medium, salting lightly. Stir frequently until the green beans deepen in color, but retain their crisp.

2. Remove the beans from heat and plunge into an ice bath to halt cooking.

3. In a small bowl, combine olive oil, parsley, garlic powder, salt, pepper, oregano, and pepper flakes. Stir to combine thoroughly.

4. In a large mixing bowl, combine all remaining ingredients and mix completely.

5. Drizzle dressing over the mixture and stir once more to coat.

6. Cover and chill for at least 15 minutes before serving.

7. Serve chilled!

Thai-Inspired Chicken Salad

Number of Servings: 8 | Prep Time: 10 min. | Cook Time: 0 min.

Calories: 152 | Carbohydrates: 2g | Fat: 8g | Protein: 18g | Sugar: 1g

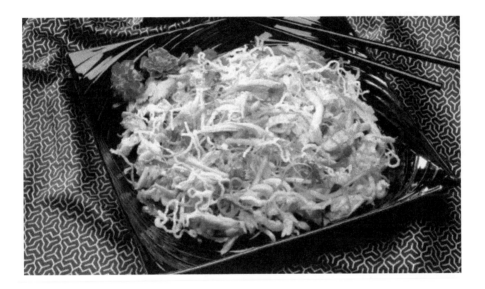

Ingredients:

¼ c. cilantro, finely chopped

¼ c. green onion, chopped

½ peanuts, roasted & unsalted

½ tsp. red pepper flakes

1 c. plain yogurt

1 med. bell pepper, diced

2 c. red cabbage, chopped

2 chicken breasts, cooked and shredded

2 tbsp. maple syrup

3 tbsp. rice wine vinegar

Sea salt & pepper to taste

Instructions:

1. In a large mixing bowl, combine all ingredients and stir to combine thoroughly.

2. Cover and chill for at least 15 minutes before serving.

3. Serve chilled!

Greek Quinoa Salad

Number of Servings: 6 | Prep Time: 10 min. | Cook Time: 15 min.

Calories: 344 | Carbohydrates: 28g | Fat: 23g | Protein: 8g |

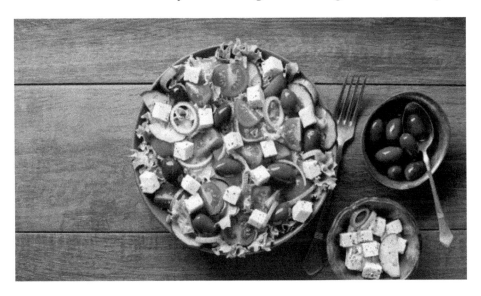

Sugar: 3g

Ingredients:

¼ c. red onion, finely chopped

½ c. feta cheese crumbles

½ c. parsley, finely chopped

½ English cucumber, chopped

1 c. quinoa, cooked according to package instructions and cooled

1 lemon, juiced

1 lg. bell pepper, chopped

1 med. tomato, diced

1 tbsp. cumin

2 tbsp. extra virgin olive oil

20 Kalamata olives pitted and halved

Sea salt & pepper, to taste

Instructions:

1. In a large mixing bowl, combine all ingredients and stir to combine thoroughly.

2. Cover and chill for at least 15 minutes before serving.

3. Serve chilled!

Dinner Recipes

Instant Pot Teriyaki Chicken

Number of Servings: 6 | Prep Time: 10 min. | Cook Time: 20 min.

Calories: 244 | Carbohydrates: 15g | Fat: 4g | Protein: 34g | Sugar: 11g

Ingredients:

¼ c. soy sauce or Bragg's Liquid Aminos

1 ½ tsp. ginger paste

1 c. water

1/3 c. honey

2 cloves garlic, minced

2 lbs. chicken breasts, boneless & skinless

2 med. green onions, sliced

3 tbsp. rice wine vinegar

For slurry:

¼ c. cold water

3 tbsp. cornstarch

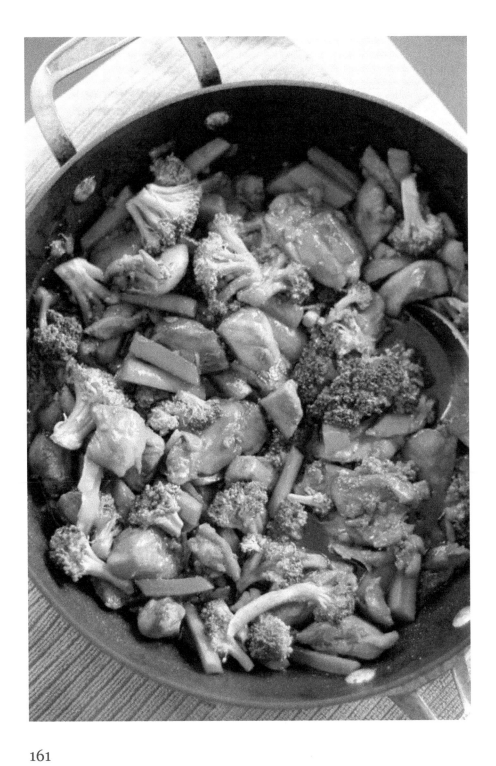

Instructions:

1. Place the Instant Pot insert into the cooker and pour water, honey, soy sauce, vinegar, garlic, and ginger. Stir to incorporate, then lay the chicken breasts on top of the liquid.

2. Seal the pressure lock and ensure the vent is also sealed. Set your cooker to high for 10 minutes.

3. Once the cooker beeps, release the pressure completely, then open the lid,

4. Shred the chicken completely using two forks or a stand mixer, then return the chicken to the pot and switch the pot to the sauté setting.

5. Mix your slurry in a small bowl, making sure there are no starch lumps in it, then pour it over the chicken.

6. Stir the chicken to incorporate the slurry, as this will thicken your sauce. Allow it to cook for a few minutes more, stirring occasionally until the sauce has reached the desired level of thickness.

7. Serve over rice, salads, quinoa, or whatever you prefer!

Chicken Tetrazzini

Number of Servings: 8 | Prep Time: 15 min. | Cook Time: 25 min.

Calories: 421 | Carbohydrates: 51g | Fat: 13g | Protein: 26g | Sugar: 8g

Ingredients:

¼ c. parmesan cheese, grated

1 c. mozzarella cheese, shredded

1 lb. chicken breast, boneless, skinless, & cubed

1 lb. whole wheat spaghetti noodles

1 med. onion, diced

1 tsp. oregano, dried

10 oz. button mushrooms, sliced

2 c. milk

2 med. bell peppers, diced

2 tbsp. extra virgin olive oil

3 c. chicken broth

3 lg. stalks celery, diced

3 tbsp. breadcrumbs

Sea salt & pepper, to taste

Instructions:

1. Warm a large pot or Dutch oven over medium heat and warm the oil in it.

2. Combine celery and onion into the pot, stirring completely to combine and allowing to cook for about three minutes or until shiny.

3. Stir the salt, pepper, mushrooms, peppers, and oregano into the pot and stir occasionally until all ingredients get shiny and begin to cook through.

4. Stir broth, milk, parmesan cheese, and chicken into the pot and stir until completely combined.

5. Break pasta noodles in half and stir them into the mixture, doing your best to get them spread evenly throughout the pot.

6. Cover and allow to cook for about ten minutes.

7. In a medium mixing bowl, combine mozzarella and breadcrumbs, mixing completely.

8. Uncover the pot and stir once more before sprinkling the cheese and crumb mixture on top. Cover and let cook for

about three to five more minutes, or until the cheese is nice and bubbly.

9. Serve hot!

Sheet Pan Steak Fajitas

Number of Servings: 4 | Prep Time: 10 min. | Cook Time: 25 min.

Calories: 555 | Carbohydrates: 47g | Fat: 23g | Protein: 39g | Sugar: 7g

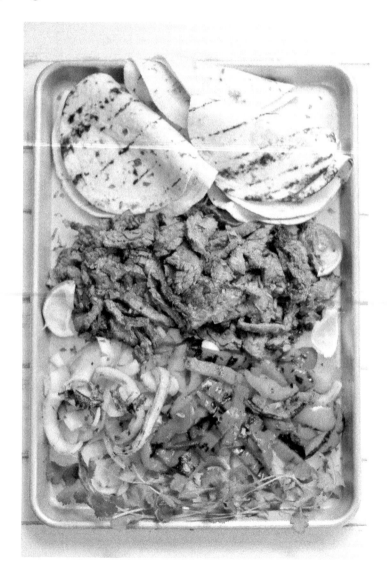

Ingredients:

For the Steak:

½ jalapeño, seeded & finely diced

½ tsp. taco seasoning

1 ½ lbs. flank steak, sliced

1 lime, juiced

1 tbsp. extra virgin olive oil

1 tsp. garlic powder

Sea salt & pepper, to taste

For the Veggies:

½ tsp. taco seasoning

2 lg. onions, thinly sliced

2 tbsp. extra virgin olive oil

3 lg. bell peppers, thinly sliced

Sea salt & pepper, to taste

To Serve:

½ c. sour cream

1 sm. avocado, finely diced

2 tbsp. cilantro, fresh & finely chopped

8 oz. sharp cheddar cheese, shredded

8 small tortillas

Lime wedges

Instructions:

1. Preheat the oven to 475° Fahrenheit and line two large baking sheets with non-stick foil.

2. Place the meat into one large mixing bowl, and the vegetables into another.

3. In the mixing bowl with the steak, combine lime juice, taco seasoning, garlic powder, salt, and pepper. Mix completely with tongs or your hands to coat the meat completely in the juice and seasonings.

4. In the mixing bowl with the vegetables, drizzle olive oil, taco seasoning, salt, and pepper. Use hands or tongs to coat completely.

5. Pour half of each bowl onto each baking sheet, then mix thoroughly with your hands so you have two pans filled with identical mixtures.

6. Try to even out the items on the baking pan so they're in one even layer.

7. Bake for 20 minutes or until the steak has reached the desired level of doneness.

8. Broil for 5 minutes to add a little bit of crisp to the meat, then pull sheets out of the oven.

9. Season fajita mixture according to taste, if needed.

10. Serve two fajitas per person!

Instant Pot Meatballs

Number of Servings: 6 | Prep Time: 10 min. | Cook Time: 10 min.

Calories: 118 | Carbohydrates: 1g | Fat: 6g | Protein: 15g | Sugar: <1g

Ingredients:

½ tbsp. balsamic vinegar

½ tsp. oregano, dried

1 lb. turkey or beef, ground

1 lg. egg

2 lg. cloves garlic, minced

2 tbsp. onion powder

15 oz. low-carb tomato sauce

Sea salt & pepper, to taste

Instructions:

1. In a large mixing bowl, combine ground meat, onion powder, garlic, oregano, salt, and pepper. Mix completely with your hands.

2. Using a small spoon or scoop, mold the meat into about 30 balls.

3. Pour the tomato sauce into the bottom of the instant pot insert and drop the meatballs into the pot one at a time. It's okay if they overlap!

4. Seal the pressure lock and ensure the pressure valve is sealed. Cook on high for seven minutes.

5. Once the timer beeps, release the pressure completely before opening the lid.

6. Stir to get the tomato sauce all over the meatballs, then serve!

Sheet Pan Chicken and Veggie Bake

Number of Servings: 8 | Prep Time: 15 min. | Cook Time: 25 min.

Calories: 421 | Carbohydrates: 51g | Fat: 13g | Protein: 26g | Sugar: 8g

Ingredients:

¼ c. parmesan cheese, grated

1 c. mozzarella cheese, shredded

1 lb. chicken breast, boneless, skinless, & cubed

1 lb. whole wheat spaghetti noodles

1 med. onion, diced

1 tsp. oregano, dried

10 oz. button mushrooms, sliced

2 c. milk

2 med. bell peppers, diced

2 tbsp. extra virgin olive oil

3 c. chicken broth

3 lg. stalks celery, diced

3 tbsp. breadcrumbs

Sea salt & pepper, to taste

Instructions:

1. Warm a large pot or Dutch oven over medium heat and warm the oil in it.

2. Combine celery and onion into the pot, stirring completely to combine and allowing to cook for about three minutes or until shiny.

3. Stir the salt, pepper, mushrooms, peppers, and oregano into the pot and stir occasionally until all ingredients get shiny and begin to cook through.

4. Stir broth, milk, parmesan cheese, and chicken into the pot and stir until completely combined.

5. Break pasta noodles in half and stir them into the mixture, doing your best to get them spread evenly throughout the pot.

6. Cover and allow to cook for about ten minutes.

7. In a medium mixing bowl, combine mozzarella and breadcrumbs, mixing completely.

8. Uncover the pot and stir once more before sprinkling the cheese and crumb mixture on top. Cover and let cook for about three to five more minutes, or until the cheese is nice and bubbly.

Black Bean & Quinoa Casserole

Number of Servings: 9 | Prep Time: 10 min. | Cook Time: 40 min.

Calories: 418 | Carbohydrates: 35g | Fat: 23g | Protein: 26g | Sugar: 4g

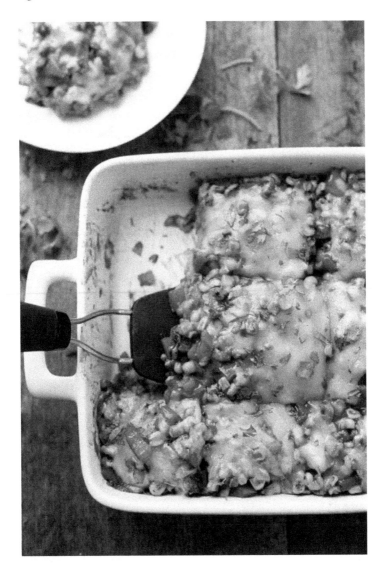

Ingredients:

½ med. jalapeño, seeded & diced

¾ c. canned coconut milk

1 ½ c. cheddar cheese, shredded

1 ½ c. corn, drained

1 tbsp. cumin

15 oz. black beans, rinsed & drained

2 cloves garlic, crushed

2 med. green onions, sliced

2 tbsp. cilantro, fresh & finely chopped

2 tbsp. extra virgin olive oil

3 c. quinoa, cooked according to package instructions and cooled

3 lg. bell peppers, diced

Sea salt & pepper, to taste

For Topping:

½ c. cheddar cheese, shredded

1 med. green onion, sliced

1 tsp. cilantro, fresh & finely chopped

Instructions:

1. Heat a large skillet over medium heat and warm the olive oil in it.

2. Preheat oven to 350° Fahrenheit and oil a baking dish.

3. Add the garlic to the skillet, allow to cook until fragrant, about 30 seconds.

4. Combine the corn, bell peppers, cumin, and jalapeño into the skillet and stir to mix the ingredients thoroughly. Cook for about three minutes, stir, then allow to cook for three minutes more.

5. In a large mixing bowl, combine cooked quinoa, vegetable mix, beans, cilantro, green onion, cheese, coconut milk, and salt. Mix well and transfer into oiled baking dish, pressing everything into an even layer.

6. Top with remaining cheese, then bake for 30 minutes.

7. Top with cilantro and green onions, and serve!

Lentil Casserole

Number of Servings: 8 | Prep Time: 10 min. | Cook Time: 70 min.

Calories: 267 | Carbohydrates: 35g | Fat: 9g | Protein: 15g | Sugar: 5g

Ingredients:

½ tsp. thyme

1 ½ c. green lentils, rinsed

1 lb. brown mushrooms, sliced

1 lg. onion, diced

1 tsp. garlic powder

12 oz. cream of mushroom soup

2 c. water, boiled

2 lg. carrots, diced

3 lg. stalks celery, diced

3 tbsp. extra virgin olive oil

4 oz. mozzarella cheese, shredded

Sea salt & pepper to taste

Instructions:

1. Preheat oven to 375° Fahrenheit and oil a large baking dish with cooking spray or oil of your preference.

2. Over medium heat, preheat a medium skillet with olive oil in it.

3. Add onion, celery, and carrots to the skillet and allow to cook for about five minutes, stirring throughout. Empty the skillet into the baking dish, then return the skillet to the heat with more olive oil.

4. Kick the heat up to high and add the mushrooms to the skillet. Let them brown a little bit, then add them into the baking dish.

5. Return the skillet to the heat once more, dropping the heat down to low. Add oil, garlic powder, and thyme to the skillet, stir thoroughly, then add the lentils. Let that heat through for about two minutes, then add the water to the skillet.

6. While the water comes to a boil, use your spatula to light graze the bottom of the skillet to loosen the fond that has accumulated there.

7. Once boiling, add the soup to the pan and stir completely, adding more sea salt and pepper as is needed. Kill the heat and scrape the mixture into the baking dish. Thoroughly incorporate all ingredients in the dish and smooth it into one even layer.

8. Cover the dish with foil and bake for 30 minutes.

9. Remove the foil and return the dish to the oven for another 15 minutes.

10. Sprinkle cheese on top of the casserole, then return to the oven for up to five minutes or until the cheese is bubbly.

11. Let stand about 20 minutes to allow the dish to firm up, then serve hot!

Cheeseburger Quinoa Casserole

Number of Servings: 8 | Prep Time: 5 min. | Cook Time: 75 min.

Calories: 261 | Carbohydrates: 30g | Fat: 6g | Protein: 22g | Sugar: 6g

Ingredients:

1 ¼ c. quinoa, dry

1 c. tomato sauce

1 lb. ground turkey

1 med. onion, diced

1 tbsp. yellow mustard

1 tsp. extra virgin olive oil

1 tsp. Worcestershire sauce

12 oz. cream of mushroom soup

2 c. chicken broth

2 cloves garlic, minced

2 lg. bell peppers, diced

3 med. tomatoes, diced

4 oz. cheddar cheese, shredded & divided

Sea salt & pepper, to taste

Instructions:

1. Preheat oven to 400° Fahrenheit and oil a large baking dish with oil or non-stick spray of your preference.

2. Heat a large skillet over medium heat and add olive oil to prevent sticking. Sauté onion, garlic, and peppers until just translucent, then transfer into a large mixing bowl.

3. Return the skillet to the stove over medium-high heat and brown the ground meat, breaking into pieces as you do so. Once cooked, transfer the cooked meat into the large mixing bowl along with all the remaining ingredients, except half of the cheese.

4. Stir the mixture completely until everything is fully incorporated, then transfer to the baking dishes, spreading everything evenly into one layer.

5. Cover the dish with foil and bake for 40 minutes, then top with the remaining cheese. Return to the oven uncovered and allow to cook for another five to ten minutes, or until the cheese bubbly.

6. Serve hot!

TIP: If you're a sucker for burger sauce like I am, mix 1 tbsp. mayo, ½ tbsp. sugar-free ketchup, ½ tbsp. yellow mustard, ½ tbsp. dill relish with a little bit of garlic powder and voila! Top your casserole and enjoy!

Teriyaki Salmon

Number of Servings: 6 | Prep Time: 10 min. | Cook Time: 20 min.

Calories: 212 | Carbohydrates: 7g | Fat: 7g | Protein: 32g | Sugar: 6g

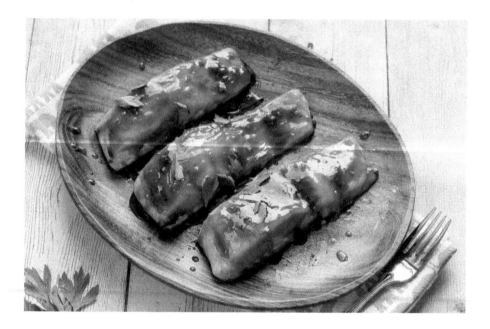

Ingredients:

24 oz. salmon fillets, sliced into 4 oz. strips

3 tbsp. honey

2 tbsp. soy sauce

1 tbsp. rice wine vinegar

1 clove garlic, minced

½ tsp. ginger paste

2 med. green onions, sliced

For the Slurry:

2 tbsp. cold water

1 tsp. cornstarch

Instructions:

1. In a small bowl, combine honey, ginger, garlic, soy sauce, and vinegar. Mix thoroughly with a fork and pour the sauce into a baking dish.

2. Place the pieces of salmon in the dish, coating each piece in the sauce, leaving them in it, pink-side-down until the oven is fully preheated.

3. Preheat oven to 450° Fahrenheit and line a large baking sheet with non-stick foil.

4. Once the oven is preheated, lie the salmon pieces on the foil skin-side-down, making sure to leave a bit of room in between each piece.

5. In a small pot on the stove, warm the leftover marinade over medium heat. In another small bowl, mix the slurry together, then when there are no lumps left in it, stir it into the sauce in the pot and stir continuously until it thickens.

6. Allow the salmon to bake for 15-20 minutes or until it's just done enough.

7. Remove the salmon from the oven and coat with the glaze, topping with sesame seeds and sliced green onions to preference.

8. Serve hot!

Cheesy Pasta Bake

Number of Servings: 8 | Prep Time: 10 min. | Cook Time: 40 min.

Calories: 355 | Carbohydrates: 41g | Fat: 4g | Protein: 43g | Sugar: 11g

Ingredients:

1 c. pasta water

1 lg. cloves garlic, minced

1 lg. onion, diced

1 tbsp. Italian seasoning, dried

1 tsp. extra virgin olive oil

2 lbs. turkey, ground

3 c. whole wheat penne pasta, al dente

3 tbsp. parsley, fresh & finely chopped

5 c. kale, chopped & de-stemmed

8 oz. mozzarella cheese, shredded & divided

28 oz. tomato sauce

Sea salt & pepper, to taste

Instructions:

1. Preheat oven to 375° Fahrenheit and oil a large baking dish with non-stick spray or your choice of oil.

2. In a large skillet over medium heat, sauté onion and garlic until shiny and fragrant, then add ground meat. Brown the meat and break it up into chunks as you do so.

3. Add remaining ingredients including pasta—except for cheese—into the skillet and mix completely.

4. Kill the heat and pour half the mixture into the casserole dish, topping with half of the shredded cheese.

5. Pour the second half of the mix into the casserole dish and top with remaining cheese.

6. Cover with foil and bake for 25 minutes. Remove foil and allow to bake uncovered until the cheese has browned nicely.

7. Serve hot!

Snack Recipes

Apple Bread

Number of Servings: 10 | Prep Time: 20 min. | Cook Time: 60 min.

Calories: 210 | Carbohydrates: 41g | Fat: 5g | Protein: 5g | Sugar: 17g

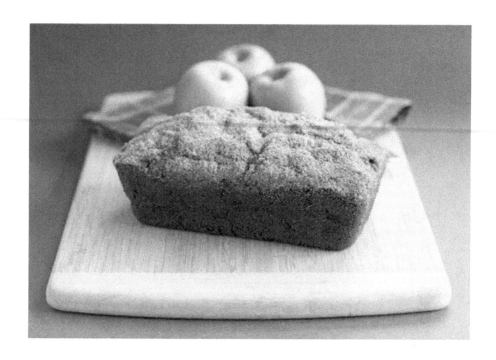

Ingredients:

½ c. honey

½ tsp. nutmeg

½ tsp. salt

1 c. applesauce, sweetened

1 tsp. baking soda

1 tsp. vanilla extract

2 ¼ c. whole wheat flour

2 lg. eggs

2 tbsp. vegetable oil (or preferred oil)

2 tsp. baking powder

2 tsp. cinnamon

4 c. apples, diced

Instructions:

1. Preheat oven to 375° Fahrenheit and oil a loaf pan with non-stick spray or your choice of oil.

2. In a large mixing bowl, beat eggs until completely smooth.

3. Add the honey, oil, applesauce, cinnamon, vanilla, nutmeg, baking powder, baking soda, and salt. Whisk until completely combined and smooth.

4. Add the flour into the bowl and whisk to combine, making sure not to over-mix. Simply stir it enough to incorporate the flour.

5. Add apples to the batter and mix once more to combine.

6. Pour the batter into the loaf pan and smooth the top with your spatula.

7. Bake for 60 minutes, or until an inserted toothpick in the center comes out clean.

8. Let stand for 10 minutes, then transfer the loaf to a cooling rack to cool completely.

9. Slice into 10 pieces and serve!

Coconut Protein Balls

Number of Servings: 27 | Prep Time: 20 min. | Cook Time: 0 min.

Calories: 108 | Carbohydrates: 16g | Fat: 4g | Protein: 5g | Sugar: 13g

Ingredients:

¼ c. dark chocolate chips

½ c. coconut flakes, unsweetened

½ c. water

1 ½ c. almonds, raw & unsalted

2 tbsp. cocoa powder, unsweetened

3 c. Medjool dates, pitted

4 scoops whey protein powder, unsweetened

Instructions:

1. Process almonds in a food processor until a flour is formed. Add the water and dates to the flour and continue to process until fully combined. You may need to stop intermittently to scrape down the sides of the bowl.

2. Add cocoa and protein to the processor and continue to process until well combined. You may need to stop intermittently to scrape down the sides of the bowl.

3. Pull the blade out of the processor (carefully!) and use your spatula to gather all of the dough in one place inside the processor container.

4. On a plate or in a large, shallow dish, spread the coconut flakes.

5. Using a spoon, scoop out a little bit of the dough at a time and roll it into balls, then roll each one in the coconut flakes.

6. Refrigerate for at least 30 min before enjoying.

These can be refrigerated for up to one week, or frozen for up to three months!

Carrot Muffins

Number of Servings: 12 | Prep Time: 10 min. | Cook Time: 25 min.

Calories: 137 | Carbohydrates: 26g | Fat: 4g | Protein: 5g | Sugar: 10g

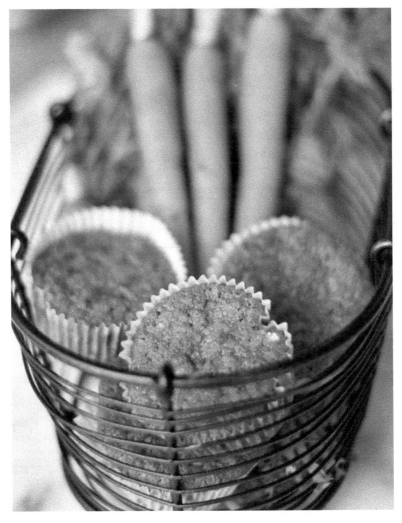

Ingredients:

⅓ c. raisins

⅓ c. walnuts, chopped

½ tsp. nutmeg

½ tsp. salt

¾ c. applesauce, unsweetened

¾ tsp. baking soda

1 ½ c. carrots, grated

1 c. quick oats

1 c. wheat flour

1 tsp. cinnamon

1 tsp. vanilla extract

1/3 c. honey

2 lg. eggs

2 tsp. baking powder

Instructions:

1. Preheat oven to 375° Fahrenheit and oil a muffin tin with non-stick spray or your choice of oil.

2. In a large mixing bowl, whisk eggs. Add applesauce, honey, vanilla, cinnamon, nutmeg, baking soda, baking powder, and salt. Whisk to combine.

3. Add the carrots to the mixture and stir completely.

4. Add the flour and oats and stir just until combined.

5. Stir nuts and raisins into the mix and stir until combined.

6. Pour or spoon the batter into each of the 12 wells in the muffin tins and bake for about 25 minutes or until a toothpick inserted into the middle of the middlemost muffin comes out clean.

7. Let stand for about 10 minutes before transferring muffins to a cooling rack to cool completely.

8. Enjoy!

Chocolate Chia Pudding

Number of Servings: 1 | Prep Time: 3 min. | Chill Time: 6 hr.

Calories: 329 | Carbohydrates: 40g | Fat: 14g | Protein: 14g | Sugar: 18g

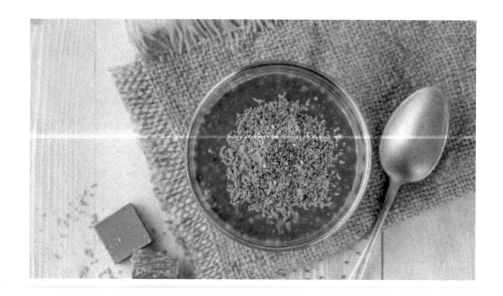

Ingredients:

¾ c. milk, unsweetened

2 tsp. honey

1 tsp. vanilla extract

4 tbsp. chia seeds

1 tbsp. cocoa powder, unsweetened

Instructions:

1. In a glass jar or container, combine all liquid ingredients and mix completely.

2. Add chia seeds and cocoa powder and mix completely.

3. Allow everything to sit for about 10 minutes before stirring once again, then sealing tightly and storing in the refrigerator overnight.

4. Stir well before eating and enjoy cold!

Blueberry Muffins

Number of Servings: 12 | Prep Time: 5 min. | Cook Time: 25 min.

Calories: 329 | Carbohydrates: 40g | Fat: 14g | Protein: 14g | Sugar: 18g

Ingredients:

¼ c. vegetable oil (or preferred oil)

¼ tsp. salt

½ tsp. baking soda

1 ½ c. blueberries, frozen

1 c. applesauce, unsweetened

1 tsp. cinnamon

1 tsp. vanilla extract

1/3 c. honey

2 c. whole wheat flour

2 lg. eggs, beaten

2 tsp. baking powder

Instructions:

1. Preheat oven to 350° Fahrenheit and line a muffin tin with paper liners.

2. In a large mixing bowl, combine eggs, apple sauce, honey, oil, vanilla extract, cinnamon, baking soda, salt, and baking powder. Whisk until completely combined, ensuring that there are no lumps of baking powder or soda.

3. Add flour to the batter and whisk until just combined.

4. Add blueberries and mix.

5. Fill the muffin tins and bake for 22-25 minutes or until a toothpick inserted into the middle of the middlemost muffin comes out clean.

6. Let cool for 30 minutes before transferring to a cooling rack to cool completely.

7. Serve and enjoy!

Peanut Butter Protein Bites

Number of Servings: 25 | Prep Time: 30 min. | Cook Time: 0 min.

Calories: 107 | Carbohydrates: 9g | Fat: 6g | Protein: 5g | Sugar: 4g

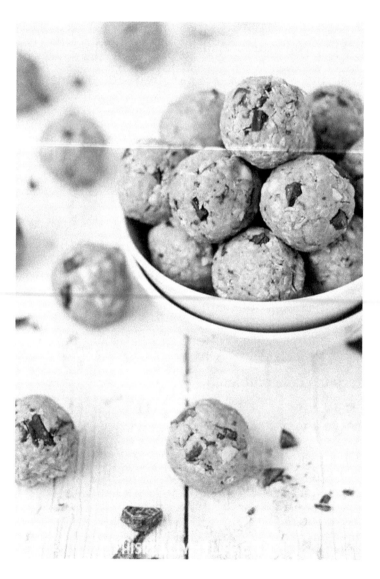

Ingredients:

¼ c. flaxseed, ground

¼ c. honey

¼ tsp. salt

1 c. peanut butter, warmed

1 c. quick oats

2 tbsp. chocolate chips

4 scoops whey protein powder

5 tbsp. water

Instructions:

1. In a mixing bowl, combine all ingredients and mix well.

2. Refrigerate the mix for 20 minutes.

3. Using a spoon or small scoop, take bits of the dough out and roll it into balls.

4. Serve!

Quinoa Protein Bars

Number of Servings: 16 | Prep Time: 15 min. | Cook Time: 40 min.

Calories: 269 | Carbohydrates: 30g | Fat: 15g | Protein: 6g | Sugar: 13g

Ingredients:

½ c. almonds, chopped

½ c. chocolate chips

½ c. coconut oil, melted

½ c. flaxseed, ground

½ c. honey

½ tsp. salt

1 c. quinoa, dry

2 ¼ c. quick oats

3 lg. egg whites

Instructions:

1. Preheat oven to 325° Fahrenheit and spread oats, quinoa, and almonds evenly in the bottom of a clean, dry baking sheet.

2. Bake for 10 to 15 minutes or until all ingredients have browned lightly. You may want to stir the items in the cookie sheet every few minutes to ensure nothing burns.

3. Remove grains and nuts from the oven and allow to cool completely, but don't turn off the oven.

4. In a large mixing bowl, whisk the egg whites and beat the coconut oil and honey into them.

5. Combine flaxseed, chocolate chips, and salt into the cooled grains and nuts and then pour that mixture into the mixing bowl, coating everything completely.

6. Line your baking sheet with parchment paper and spread the mixture evenly onto it, pressing it into one even layer. You may want to shape the sides of the mass, depending on whether or not it reaches the edges of your baking sheet without thinning out too much.

7. Bake for 30 minutes, then remove from the oven.

8. Let cool for one hour before slicing into evenly-shaped bars, then cool completely.

9. Enjoy!

Protein Bars

Number of Servings: 12 | Prep Time: 10 min. | Cook Time: 30 min.

Calories: 186 | Carbohydrates: 7g | Fat: 14g | Protein: 8g | Sugar: 4g

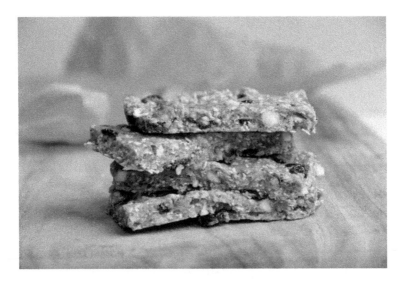

Ingredients:

For the bars:

$^{1/3}$ c. coconut oil

$^{1/3}$ c. creamy peanut butter, unsalted

$^{1/3}$ c. almond meal

½ c. milk of your choice, unsweetened

1 ½ c. protein powder

For the Topping:

2 tbsp. chocolate chips

1 tbsp. coconut oil

3 tbsp. almonds, chopped

Instructions:

1. In a microwave-safe bowl, combine peanut butter, milk and all but one tablespoon of the coconut oil. Heat for 30-second intervals, stirring in between, until completely smooth.

2. Mix almond meal and protein powder into the bowl and combine well until a crumbly dough is combined.

3. Line a baking dish with parchment paper and flatten the dough into it until an even layer is formed.

4. In a small, microwave-safe bowl, combine the chocolate chips and 1 tbsp. of coconut oil and heat for 30-second intervals, stirring in between until completely smooth.

5. Pour the chocolate mixture over the bars and spread it evenly. Sprinkle the almonds on top and then freeze the bars for about 20 minutes, or refrigerate them for about an hour.

6. Cut into 12 evenly-shaped bars and enjoy!

Tropical Chia Pudding

Number of Servings: 1 | Prep Time: 1 min. | Chill Time: 6 hr.

Calories: 269 | Carbohydrates: 30g | Fat: 15g | Protein: 6g | Sugar: 13g

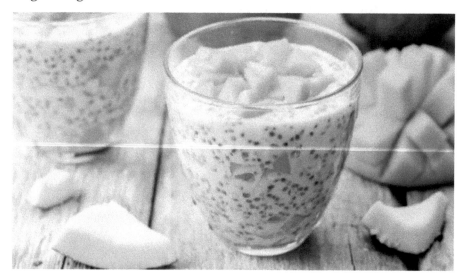

Ingredients:

¼ c. chia seeds

½ c. almond milk, vanilla & unsweetened

1 c. coconut milk, light

1 c. fresh mango, chopped

1 tsp. coconut flakes, unsweetened

Instructions:

1. Combine all ingredients into a glass container with a lid and stir completely.

2. Refrigerate for six to eight hours.

3. Stir and serve chilled!

Oh-So-Easy Strawberry Smoothie

Number of Servings: 2 | Prep Time: 5 min. | Cook Time: 0 min.

Calories: 180 | Carbohydrates: 32g | Fat: 6g | Protein: 4g | Sugar: 15g

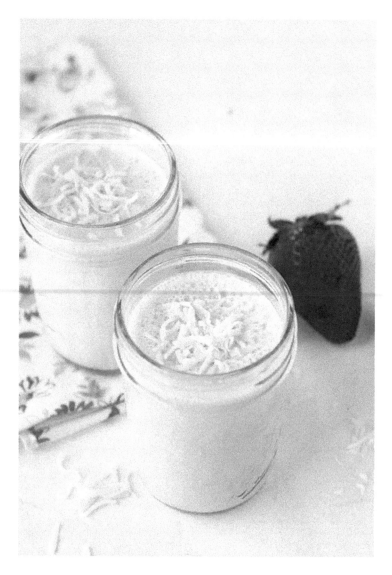

Ingredients:

½ c. almonds, chopped

1 ½ c. almond milk, unsweetened

1 lg. banana, ripe

2 c. strawberries, frozen

2 tbsp. flaxseed, ground

Instructions:

1. Roughly chop banana into chunks.

2. Combine all ingredients into the blender, adding the milk first.

3. Blend until smooth.

4. Serve cold!

Conclusion

Thank you for reading *Intermittent Fasting for Women over 50: The Ultimate Guide for a Natural Approach to Weight Loss and Looking Younger, Formulated for Mature Women*. May the information that you've read in these chapters guide you and advise you in achieving your goals, whatever they may be.

If you haven't set any health and wellness goals with the information that you've learned here, your next step would be to do so! Set some goals for yourself that you can comfortably achieve and start making steps toward a more healthful and beneficial regimen that you can comfortably stick to.

If you're someone who likes to jump right into a new path or regimen, pick the intermittent fasting schedule that works best for you, or which sounds most appealing to you and get started as soon as you can.

Take the recipes from this book that appeal to you and your tastes the most and craft your shopping list that will get you on your way to doing the most for yourself and your body. You will find that some of the recipes in this book have some places where you can make some substitutions, so be sure that you take a look at all the ingredients and choose the ones that work best for you and which make you feel your best!

It will never be our suggestion that you hold yourself to using things like dairy or nut products if you have allergies, or if you simply feel better when using alternatives, so feel free to substitute any ingredients you wish and to create your own recipes using these ones as a starting point!

Finally, if you found the information and resources in this book to be helpful to you in getting started on the right path, then an Amazon review would be greatly appreciated!

CPSIA information can be obtained
at www.ICGtesting.com
Printed in the USA
LVHW051441300321
682937LV00019B/995